Parkinson Disease

Editors

CARLOS SINGER
STEPHEN G. REICH

CLINICS IN
GERIATRIC MEDICINE

www.geriatric.theclinics.com

February 2020 • Volume 36 • Number 1

ELSEVIER

1600 John F. Kennedy Boulevard • Suite 1800 • Philadelphia, Pennsylvania, 19103-2899

http://www.theclinics.com

CLINICS IN GERIATRIC MEDICINE Volume 36, Number 1
February 2020 ISSN 0749–0690, ISBN-13: 978-0-323-69818-4

Editor: Katerina Heidhausen
Developmental Editor: Laura Fisher

Clinics in Geriatric Medicine (ISSN 0749-0690) is published quarterly by Elsevier Inc., 360 Park Avenue South, New York, NY 10010-1710. Months of issue are February, May, August, and November. Business and Editorial Offices: 1600 John F. Kennedy Blvd., Suite 1800, Philadelphia, PA 191023-2899. Periodicals postage paid at New York, NY, and additional mailing offices. Subscription prices are $289.00 per year (US individuals), $664.00 per year (US institutions), $100.00 per year (US & Canadian student/resident), $320.00 per year (Canadian individuals), $841.00 per year (Canadian institutions), $414.00 per year (international individuals), $841.00 per year (international institutions), and $195.00 per year (international student/resident). Foreign air speed delivery is included in all *Clinics* subscription prices. All prices are subject to change without notice. POSTMASTER: Send address changes to *Clinics in Geriatric Medicine,* Elsevier Health Sciences Division, Subscription Customer Service, 3251 Riverport Lane, Maryland Heights, MO 63043. **Telephone: 1-800-654-2452 (U.S. and Canada); 314-447-8871 (outside U.S. and Canada). Fax: 314-447-8029. E-mail:** journalscustomerservice-usa@elsevier.com **(for print support)** or journalsonlinesupport-usa@elsevier.com **(for online support).**

Reprints. For copies of 100 or more, of articles in this publication, please contact the Commercial Reprints Department, Elsevier Inc., 360 Park Avenue South, New York, New York 10010-1710. Tel.: 212-633-3874; Fax: 212-633-3820, E-mail: reprints@elsevier.com.

Clinics in Geriatric Medicine is covered in *MEDLINE/PubMed (Index Medicus), EMBASE/Excerpta Medica, Current Contents/Clinical Medicine (CC/CM),* and the *Cumulative Index to Nursing & Allied Health Literature.*

Contributors

EDITORS

CARLOS SINGER, MD
Professor of Neurology, Chief, Division of Parkinson Disease and Movement Disorders, University of Miami Miller School of Medicine, Miami, Florida, USA

STEPHEN G. REICH, MD
Professor of Neurology, The Frederick Henry Prince Distinguished Professor in Neurology, Department of Neurology, University of Maryland School of Medicine, Baltimore, Maryland, USA

AUTHORS

PINKY AGARWAL, MD, FAAN
Booth Gardner Parkinson's Care Center, Evergreen Neuroscience Institute, Kirkland, Washington, USA; Clinical Professor, University of Washington, Seattle, Washington, USA

SAGARI BETTÉ, MD
Department of Neurology, Instructor, University of Miami Miller School of Medicine, Miami, Florida, USA; Neurologist, Parkinson Disease and Movement Disorders Center of Boca Raton, Boca Raton, Florida, USA

YAREMA BEZCHLIBNYK, MD, PhD
University of South Florida, Movement Disorders Neuromodulation Center, Department of Neurosurgery and Brain Repair, University of South Florida, Tampa, Florida, USA

BASTIAAN R. BLOEM, MD, PhD
Department of Neurology, Radboud University Medical Centre, Donders Institute for Brain, Cognition and Behaviour, Nijmegen, The Netherlands

PATRIK BRUNDIN, MD, PhD
Associate Director, Van Andel Research Institute, Director, Center for Neurodegenerative Science, Van Andel Institute, Grand Rapids, Michigan, USA

STEFANO CAPRONI, MD, PhD
Neurology Division, Neuroscience Department, "S. Maria" University Hospital, Terni, Italy

LESLIE JAMELEH CLOUD, MD, MSc
VCU NOW Center, Henrico, Virginia, USA; Associate Professor of Neurology, Parkinson's and Movement Disorders Center, Virginia Commonwealth University School of Medicine, Richmond, Virginia, USA

CARLO COLOSIMO, MD, FEAN
Neurology Division, Neuroscience Department, "S. Maria" University Hospital, Terni, Italy

MARIAN LIVINGSTON DALE, MD, MCR
Assistant Professor, Department of Neurology, Oregon Health and Science University, Portland, Oregon, USA

NIENKE M. DE VRIES, PT, PhD
Department of Neurology, Radboud University Medical Centre, Donders Institute for Brain, Cognition and Behaviour, Nijmegen, The Netherlands

HANNES DEVOS, PhD
Assistant Professor, Department of Physical Therapy and Rehabilitation Science, The University of Kansas, The University of Kansas Medical Center, Kansas City, Kansas, USA

NICOLAS DOHSE, BS
Department of Neurology, University of South Florida, Ataxia Research Center, Tampa, Florida, USA; Frances J. Zesiewicz Foundation for Parkinson's Disease, Sidney Kimmel Medical College, Thomas Jefferson University, Philadelphia, Pennsylvania, USA

NICHOLAS FLEMING, MD
Resident, Department of Neurology, Virginia Commonwealth University School of Medicine, Richmond, Virginia, USA; VCU NOW Center, Henrico, Virginia, USA

SUSAN H. FOX, MRCP(UK), PhD
The Edmond J. Safra Program in Parkinson's Disease and the Morton and Gloria Shulman Movement Disorders Clinic, Division of Neurology, Department of Medicine, Toronto Western Hospital, University Health Network, University of Toronto, Krembil Research Institute, Toronto, Ontario, Canada

SHAILA D. GHANEKAR
Department of Neurology, University of South Florida, Ataxia Research Center, Frances J. Zesiewicz Foundation for Parkinson's Disease, University of South Florida, Movement Disorders Neuromodulation Center, Tampa, Florida, USA

PRITI GROS, MD
Division of Neurology, University of Toronto, St. Michael's Hospital, Toronto, Ontario, Canada

HORACIO KAUFMANN, MD
Professor, Department of Neurology, Dysautonomia Center, NYU School of Medicine, NYU Langone Health, New York, New York, USA

BENZI M. KLUGER, MS, MD
Department of Neurology, University of Colorado Denver, University of Colorado Anschutz Medical Campus, Aurora, Colorado, USA

ANTHONY E. LANG, MD
The Edmond J. Safra Program in Parkinson's Disease and the Morton and Gloria Shulman Movement Disorders Clinic, Division of Neurology, Department of Medicine, Toronto Western Hospital, University Health Network, University of Toronto, Krembil Research Institute, Toronto, Ontario, Canada

JOHN LEGGE, MD
Resident, Department of Neurology, Virginia Commonwealth University School of Medicine, Richmond, Virginia, USA; VCU NOW Center, Henrico, Virginia, USA

KARLO J. LIZARRAGA, MD, MS
The Edmond J. Safra Program in Parkinson's Disease and the Morton and Gloria Shulman Movement Disorders Clinic, Division of Neurology, Department of Medicine, Toronto Western Hospital, University Health Network, University of Toronto, Krembil Research Institute, Toronto, Ontario, Canada; Motor Physiology and Neuromodulation Program, Division of Movement Disorders, Department of Neurology, Center for Health + Technology (CHeT), University of Rochester, Rochester, New York, USA

CORNELIU C. LUCA, MD, PhD
Division of Parkinson Disease and Movement Disorders, Department of Neurology, University of Miami Miller School of Medicine, Miami, Florida, USA

HILLARY D. LUM, MD, PhD
Division of Geriatric Medicine, Department of Medicine, University of Colorado Denver, University of Colorado Anschutz Medical Campus, Eastern Colorado VA Geriatric Research Education and Clinical Center, Aurora, Colorado, USA

JASON MARGOLESKY, MD
Department of Neurology, Assistant Professor, University of Miami Miller School of Medicine, Miami, Florida, USA

HENRY MOORE, MD
Division of Parkinson Disease and Movement Disorders, Department of Neurology, University of Miami Miller School of Medicine, Miami, Florida, USA

JORIK NONNEKES, MD, PhD
Department of Rehabilitation, Radboud University Medical Centre, Donders Institute for Brain, Cognition and Behaviour, Nijmegen, The Netherlands

JOSE-ALBERTO PALMA, MD, PhD
Associate Professor, Department of Neurology, Dysautonomia Center, NYU School of Medicine, NYU Langone Health, New York, New York, USA

ADOLFO RAMIREZ-ZAMORA, MD
Associate Professor of Neurology, University of Florida, Fixel Center for Neurological Diseases, Gainesville, Florida, USA

MAUD RANCHET, PhD
Researcher, Laboratoire Ergonomie Sciences Cognitives pour les Transports (LESCOT), IFSTTAR (Institut Français des Sciences et Technologies des Transports, de l'Aménagement et des Réseaux), Lyon, Bron, France

SUDESHNA RAY, MD
Booth Gardner Parkinson's Care Center, Evergreen Neuroscience Institute, Kirkland, Washington, USA

STEPHEN G. REICH, MD
Professor of Neurology, The Frederick Henry Prince Distinguished Professor in Neurology, Department of Neurology, University of Maryland School of Medicine, Baltimore, Maryland, USA

DANIELLE S. SHPINER, MD
Division of Parkinson Disease and Movement Disorders, Department of Neurology, University of Miami Miller School of Medicine, Miami, Florida, USA

DAVID K. SIMON, MD, PhD
Professor of Neurology, Beth Israel Deaconess Medical Center, Harvard Medical School, Boston, Massachusetts, USA

CARLOS SINGER, MD
Professor of Neurology, Chief, Division of Parkinson Disease and Movement Disorders, University of Miami Miller School of Medicine, Miami, Florida, USA

ANTONIO P. STRAFELLA, MD, PhD
The Edmond J. Safra Program in Parkinson's Disease and the Morton and Gloria Shulman Movement Disorders Clinic, Division of Neurology, Department of Medicine, Toronto Western Hospital, University Health Network, University of Toronto, Krembil Research Institute, Toronto, Ontario, Canada

CAROLINE M. TANNER, MD, PhD
Professor of Neurology, University of California, San Francisco, Director, PADRECC, San Francisco VA Health Care System, San Francisco, California, USA

ANOUK TOSSERAMS, MD
Departments of Rehabilitation and Neurology, Radboud University Medical Centre, Donders Institute for Brain, Cognition and Behaviour, Nijmegen, The Netherlands

TAKASHI TSUBOI, MD, PhD
Research Fellow, Associate Professor of Neurology, University of Florida, Fixel Center for Neurological Diseases, Gainesville, Florida, USA

ERGUN Y. UC, MD
Professor, Department of Neurology, University of Iowa, University of Iowa Hospitals & Clinics, Neurology Service, VA Medical Center, Iowa City, Iowa, USA

ALEKSANDAR VIDENOVIC, MD, MSc
Movement Disorders Unit, Division of Sleep Medicine, Massachusetts General Hospital, Harvard Medical School, Neurologic Clinical Research Institute, Boston, Massachusetts, USA

THERESA A. ZESIEWICZ, MD, FAAN
Department of Neurology, University of South Florida, Ataxia Research Center, Frances J. Zesiewicz Foundation for Parkinson's Disease, University of South Florida, Movement Disorders Neuromodulation Center, Tampa, Florida, USA

Contents

Parkinson disease is a complex, age-related, neurodegenerative disease associated with dopamine deficiency and both motor and nonmotor deficits. Many environmental and genetic factors influence Parkinson disease risk, with different factors predominating in different patients. These factors converge on specific pathways, including mitochondrial dysfunction, oxidative stress, protein aggregation, impaired autophagy, and neuroinflammation. Ultimately, treatment of Parkinson disease may focus on targeted therapies for pathophysiologically defined subtypes of Parkinson disease patients.

Parkinsonism is one of the most common neurologic disorders in the aging population. Although Parkinson disease (PD) is the most common cause, there is a lengthy differential diagnosis. The diagnosis of PD hinges on recognizing its typical features, including bradykinesia, rest tremor, unilateral onset, cogwheel rigidity, and beneficial and sustained response to levodopa. Equally important is to be familiar with the "red flags," which are features not expected with PD and suggest an alternative diagnosis, usually a parkinsonian syndrome. In general, it is best to have the diagnosis confirmed by a neurologist, especially one with expertise in movement disorders.

In the elderly patient with tremor, the differential diagnosis is usually between essential tremor (ET) and Parkinson disease (PD). A careful history and examination are the keys to the diagnosis. Essential tremor is a bilateral action tremor of the upper limbs whereas PD begins unilaterally and is a rest tremor. A handwriting sample can usually distinguish PD from ET as the former is small (micrographic) but atremulous whereas writing in ET is tremulous but normal sized. In ET, there are no signs aside from tremor but in PD, the tremor is accompanied by bradykinesia and rigidity.

Early Parkinson disease is the approximate time period between initial diagnosis and the onset of motor fluctuations. Treatment requires an integrative approach, including identification of motor and nonmotor symptoms, choice of pharmacologic treatment, and emphasis on exercise. Patients should be treated for motor symptoms, whereas medications may be delayed for milder symptoms. The choice of treatment in patients with early Parkinson disease must be weighed against financial considerations, ease of administration, and potential long-term adverse events. Nonmotor symptoms should also be identified and treated. Exercise is an important component for treatment of Parkinson disease at any stage.

Advanced Parkinson disease (PD) is characterized by the presence of motor fluctuations becoming the focus of treatment, prominent postural instability, significant disability despite levodopa therapy, and the presence of symptoms refractory to levodopa therapy. In this article, the authors review the motor manifestations of patients with advanced PD, as well as the most common pharmacologic and nonpharmacologic available therapies.

Orthostatic hypotension (OH) is a sustained fall in blood pressure on standing that can cause symptoms of organ hypoperfusion. OH is associated with increased morbidity and mortality and leads to a significant number of hospital admissions. OH can be caused by volume depletion, blood loss, cardiac pump failure, large varicose veins, medications, or defective activation of sympathetic nerves and reduced norepinephrine release upon standing. Neurogenic OH is a frequent and disabling problem in patients with synucleinopathies such as Parkinson disease, multiple system atrophy, and pure autonomic failure, and it is commonly associated with supine hypertension. Several therapeutic options are available.

Parkinson disease (PD) is a complex of motor and nonmotor symptoms. Among the nonmotor symptoms, urinary and sexual dysfunctions are common and negatively affect the quality of life. More than 50% of patients with PD complain of urinary dysfunction and 20% have sexual dysfunction. Understanding the anatomy and physiology of the urogenital system informs the rationale for the mechanism of action of drug therapies. The management of urinary and sexual dysfunction in PD, including behavioral, medical, and procedural interventions, is reviewed in this article.

This article reviews the most common gastrointestinal (GI) problems that occur in patients with Parkinson disease, including weight loss, drooling, dysphagia, delayed gastric emptying, constipation, and defecatory dysfunction. Appropriate workup and treatment options are reviewed in detail in order to provide clinicians with a comprehensive and practical guide to managing these problems in Parkinson disease patients. GI adverse effects of commonly used Parkinson disease motor medications are also reviewed.

Depression and anxiety are common neuropsychiatric manifestations of Parkinson disease. However, they are often under-recognized because the somatic symptoms of depression often overlap with the motor symptoms of Parkinson disease and there is low self-reporting. Clinicians need to be vigilant about early detection and treatment of anxiety and depression in the patient with Parkinson disease. The development of new therapeutic strategies, including diet, exercise, and counseling along with antidepressants provide a holistic approach to management.

Psychotic and compulsive symptoms in Parkinson disease are highly prevalent and associated with poor outcomes and greater caregiver burden. When acute, delirium should be ruled out or treated accordingly. When chronic, comorbid systemic illnesses, dementia, and psychiatric disorders should be considered. Reduction and discontinuation of anticholinergics, amantadine, dopamine agonists, and levodopa as tolerated, as well as adjunctive clozapine or quetiapine are frequently effective to manage Parkinson disease psychosis. Pimavanserin appears effective but is not widely available, and more experience is needed. Dopamine agonist discontinuation is usually successful for impulse control disorders, but requires frequent monitoring, documentation, and caregiver involvement.

Sleep disorders are common among PD patients and affect quality of life. They are often under-recognized and under-treated. Mechanisms of sleep disorders in PD remain relatively poorly understood. Improved awareness of common sleep problems in PD. Tailored treatment and evidence for efficacy are lacking. The purpose of this review is to provide an overview and update on the most common sleep disorders in PD. We review specific features of the most common sleep disorders in PD, including insomnia, excessive daytime sleepiness, sleep-disordered breathing, restless legs syndrome, circadian rhythm disorders and REM sleep behavior disorders.

This article summarizes existing literature examining orthopedic interventions for patients with Parkinson disease (PD). It reviews complications and functional outcomes of shoulder, spine, knee, and hip surgeries in PD. Causes of fall-related fractures in PD and the risk of postoperative cognitive decline after orthopedic interventions in PD are also briefly discussed.

Driving is impaired in most patients with Parkinson disease because of motor, cognitive, and visual dysfunction. Driving impairments in Parkinson disease may increase the risk of crashes and result in early driving cessation with loss of independence. Drivers with Parkinson disease should undergo comprehensive evaluations to determine fitness to drive with periodic follow-up evaluations as needed. Research in rehabilitation of driving and automation to maintain independence of patients with Parkinson disease is in progress.

Palliative care (PC) is an approach to the care of persons affected by serious illness that focuses on reducing suffering by addressing medical, psychosocial, and spiritual needs. Persons living with Parkinson disease have PC needs that begin at the time of diagnosis and continue throughout the course of the illness including nonmotor symptom burden, caregiver distress, grief, and increased mortality. Primary PC refers to essential PC skills that may be practiced by nonpalliative medicine specialists to improve outcomes for their patients.

This review elaborates on multidisciplinary care for persons living with Parkinson disease by using gait and balance impairments as an example of a treatable target that typically necessitates an integrated approach by a range of different and complementary professional disciplines. Using the International Classification of Functioning, Disability, and Health model as a framework, the authors discuss the assessment and multidisciplinary management of reduced functional mobility due to gait and balance impairments. By doing so, they highlight the complex interplay between motor and nonmotor symptoms, and their influence on rehabilitation. They outline how multidisciplinary care for Parkinson disease can be organized.

Management of patients with Parkinson disease (PD) during inpatient hospital stays is complex and poses unique challenges for physicians and ancillary staff. Patients with PD have a high risk of complications, encephalopathy, and prolonged hospital stay. Early recognition of complications and implementation of rehabilitation strategies along with appropriate management of medications are critical to improve outcomes. Patients with PD can exhibit worsening mobility and balance, insomnia, orthostatic hypotension, multiple neuropsychiatric symptoms, and gastrointestinal dysfunction while hospitalized. This review summarizes the specific in-hospital concerns observed in patients with PD and discusses potential treatment approaches.

CLINICS IN GERIATRIC MEDICINE

THE CLINICS ARE AVAILABLE ONLINE!
Access your subscription at:
www.theclinics.com

Preface

Parkinson Disease

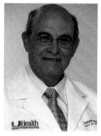 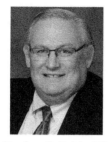

Carlos Singer, MD   Stephen G. Reich, MD
Editors

Parkinson disease (PD) is the second most prevalent neurodegenerative disorder, next only to Alzheimer disease. As the average age of the United States and European populations increases, physicians caring for the elderly will be confronted with an increasing number of PD patients.

The classic triad of tremor, rigidity, and bradykinesia allows for the diagnosis of PD in its early stages. Physicians also recognize the eventual progression to gait and balance difficulties over a period of years. Aside from applying the proper clinical criteria for diagnosis, the availability of ancillary noninvasive neuroimaging techniques assists in the early detection of the disease and decreases the period of uncertainty for patients and their families.

The recognition of levodopa as the centerpiece treatment of PD has not changed in over 50 years. What has increased is the understanding of its optimal use, its limitations, and its complications. Moreover, pharmacologic and nonpharmacologic measures have also enriched our ability to help PD patients.

However, PD is much more than a disease that affects the motor function of affected individuals. Numerous nonmotor symptoms have been identified, and they are often as, if not more, disabling than the motor features of PD, and both take a significant toll on quality of life. They span an amazing array of problems, including dysautonomia, sleep disorders, behavioral, and cognitive difficulties. There are also other issues that need to be addressed, such as the effect of the disease on orthopedic health, the decision to stop driving, the use of a multidisciplinary team approach, and the introduction of palliative medicine.

With this issue of *Clinics in Geriatric Medicine*, we have strived to provide the geriatrician, and other interested general practitioners, with information that is accessible to a general medical audience, evidence based, and relevant to daily practice. Given the limitations of publication space, "Cognitive Impairment and Dementia in

Clin Geriatr Med 36 (2020) xiii–xiv
https://doi.org/10.1016/j.cger.2019.10.001
0749-0690/20/© 2019 Published by Elsevier Inc.

Parkinson Disease" by Drs. Jennifer G. Goldman and Erica Sieg will be published in the May 2020 issue.

We wish our geriatrician colleagues all the best in the management of this challenging albeit very treatable disease.

Carlos Singer, MD
Division of Parkinson Disease and Movement Disorders
Leonard M. Miller School of Medicine
University of Miami
1150 NW 14th Street, Suite 609
Miami, FL 33136, USA

Stephen G. Reich, MD
Department of Neurology
University of Maryland School of Medicine
110 South Paca Street, 3rd Floor
Baltimore, MD 21201, USA

E-mail addresses:
csinger@med.miami.edu (C. Singer)
sreich@som.umaryland.edu (S.G. Reich)

Parkinson Disease Epidemiology, Pathology, Genetics, and Pathophysiology

David K. Simon, MD, PhD[a],*, Caroline M. Tanner, MD, PhD[b,c], Patrik Brundin, MD, PhD[d]

KEYWORDS

- Parkinson disease • Pathology • Epidemiology • Genetics • Pathophysiology
- Mitochondrial • Synuclein • Neuroprotection

KEY POINTS

- Parkinson disease is a complex, age-related, neurodegenerative disease associated with dopamine deficiency and both motor and nonmotor deficits.
- Many environmental and genetic factors influence Parkinson disease risk, with different factors predominating in different patients.
- These factors converge on specific pathways, including mitochondrial dysfunction, oxidative stress, protein aggregation, impaired autophagy, and neuroinflammation.
- Ultimately, treatment of Parkinson disease may focus on targeted therapies for pathophysiologically defined subtypes of patients with Parkinson disease.

INTRODUCTION

Parkinson disease (PD) is a complex, progressive, neurodegenerative disease described by James Parkinson in his 1817 publication, "Essay on the Shaking Palsy."[1] In that essay, Dr Parkinson optimistically declared that "there appears to be sufficient reason for hoping that some remedial process may ere long be discovered, by which, at least, the progress of the disease may be stopped." More than 200 years later we have yet to definitively achieve neuroprotective therapy for PD. However, there has been great progress in recent decades in understanding the molecular basis for

Funded by: NIHHYB: Grant number(s): R01AG059417 (C.M. Tanner); R01DC016519 (P. Brundin); R01NS086352 (D.K. Simon); R21NS094840 (D.K. Simon).
[a] Beth Israel Deaconess Medical Center, Harvard Medical School, 330 Brookline Avenue Boston, MA 02215, USA; [b] Department of Neurology, University of California - San Francisco, 1635 Divisadero St., Suite 520-530, San Francisco, CA 94115; [c] Parkinson's Disease Research Education and Clinical Center San Francisco Veteran's Affairs Medical Center, 4150 Clement St. (127P), San Francisco, CA 94121; [d] Center for Neurodegenerative Science, Van Andel Institute, 333 Bostwick Avenue Northeast, Grand Rapids, MI 49503-2518, USA
* Corresponding author.
E-mail address: dsimon1@bidmc.harvard.edu

neurodegeneration in PD, hopefully bringing us steadily getting closer to achieving truly disease-modifying therapies for PD.

Pathologically, PD is defined by loss of dopaminergic neurons in the substantia nigra pars compacta (SN) located in the midbrain and associated with Lewy bodies, which are cytoplasmic inclusions that include insoluble alpha-synuclein aggregates. However, PD is characterized by more widespread pathology in other brain regions and involves nondopaminergic neurons as well. The clinical diagnosis of PD is based primarily on motor features, such as a slowly progressive asymmetric resting tremor, cogwheel rigidity, and bradykinesia, although nonmotor features, which include anosmia, constipation, depression, and rapid eye movement sleep behavior disorder, can develop years before motor deficits. During later stages of the disease, additional nonmotor features, such as autonomic dysfunction, pain and cognitive decline, can appear.[2]

NEUROPATHOLOGY

The neuropathologic hallmarks of PD are the degeneration of dopaminergic neurons in the SN and intraneuronal protein aggregates called Lewy bodies and Lewy neurites.[3] It was long considered that 50% to 70% of SN dopaminergic neurons have died by the time that clinical motor symptoms become evident.[4] However, more recent work suggests that the loss of dopaminergic terminals in the striatum, as opposed to loss of the neurons in the SN, is crucial for onset of motor symptoms.[5]

EPIDEMIOLOGY
Distribution of Disease

In estimates based on health care use, PD incidence ranges from 5 in 100,000 to more than 35 in 100,000 new cases yearly.[6] The incidence increases by 5- to 10-fold from the sixth to the ninth decades of life. PD prevalence also increases with age. In a meta-analysis of 4 North American populations, the prevalence increased from less than 1% of men and women aged 45 to 54 years to 4% of men and 2% of women aged 85 or older.[5] Mortality is not increased, compared with nonaffected individuals in the first decade after PD is diagnosed, but increases thereafter.[7] As the global population ages, PD prevalence is expected to increase dramatically, doubling in the next 2 decades.[8] Accompanying this increase, the societal and economic burden of PD will escalate, unless more effective treatments, cures or means of prevention are identified.[9]

Determinants of Disease

Most PD cases likely have a multifactorial etiology, resulting from the combined effects of environmental and genetic factors. Exposure to toxicant chemicals and head injury may increase the risk of PD, whereas certain lifestyle factors may lower risk. Genetic susceptibility factors may modify the effects of environmental exposures. Although identifiable mutations in certain genes cause PD in around 5% to 10% of cases, these mutations are absent in most people with PD. Moreover, the most common PD-associated genetic mutations have incomplete penetrance, indicating that other environmental or genetic factors are involved. A study comparing concordance rates in monozygotic and dizygotic twins estimated the heritability of PD to be only 30%, suggesting that the majority of PD risk is related to environmental and behavioral factors.[10]

Toxicant Chemical Exposure

In studies spanning many decades in numerous populations worldwide, pesticide exposure, farm work or rural residence have been associated with an increased PD risk.[11] Occupational exposure as well as passive exposure owing to residence near to pesticide treated fields is associated with a greater risk of PD. Pesticides associated with PD, including paraquat, rotenone, 2,4-D, and several dithiocarbamates and organochlorines, cause experimental parkinsonism in laboratory studies, supporting the possibility that these associations reflect causal effects.[11,12] Genetically determined impairment in toxicant handling can amplify the effect of pesticide exposure on PD risk, an example of gene–environment interaction. Conversely, behaviors such as good hygiene practices or eating a healthy diet may protect against the adverse effects of pesticide exposure.[13,14] Chlorinated solvents (trichloroethylene, perchloroethylene, carbon tetrachloride), used in dry cleaning, degreasing, as an anesthetic and viscose rayon manufacturing and polychlorinated biphenyls, formerly used as coolants and lubricants, have also been associated with increased PD risk in humans and cause parkinsonism-associated toxicity in animal models.[12,15] Although some of these pesticides and toxicant chemicals are no longer in use, they are environmentally persistent, and remain common contaminants of soil and water. Others, such as trichloroethylene, have continuing applications and can be found in nearly one-third of US drinking water supplies, as well as in air, soil, food, and human breast milk.[16] Working as a welder also has been associated with greater risk of PD, possibly as the result of manganese in welding fumes.[17,18] Manganese exposure also can cause PD-like pathology in mice.[19] However, data on the association of welding with PD are mixed.[20] Exposure to other metals such as iron, and lead, has been suggested to increase risk of PD, based on experimental in vitro and in vivo studies, but human evidence remains inconclusive. Ambient total suspended particles from traffic has also been associated with an increased risk of PD,[21] possibly owing to metal exposure or to induction of inflammatory processes, but these findings have been inconsistent.

Head Injury

Mild to moderate head injury occurring decades before PD onset is associated with a higher risk of PD in most, but not in all studies.[12,22] Risk increases with the number of head injuries, and genetic susceptibility factors such as certain variants in or near the gene encoding alpha-synuclein may increase risk by 2- to 5-fold.

Lifestyle Factors

A number of lifestyle factors have been associated with reduced risk of developing PD. The most consistent association is a reduced risk of PD in cigarette smokers and, in a few studies, other tobacco users.[23,24] Longer duration and greater frequency of tobacco use confer lower risk and there is some evidence of genetic modification. Nicotine has been suggested to play a central role in this association, although a recently completed clinical study failed to detect a disease modifying effect of the nicotine patch in patients with PD. Coffee drinking and caffeine use are also associated with a lower risk of PD,[25,26] particularly in men. The effect is greatest in men with the highest levels of coffee use and may be further modified by genetic factors. Similarly, reports have shown reduced risk of PD in heavy tea drinkers in some, but not all populations studied. Conversely, greater dietary intake of dairy products has been associated with a higher risk of PD, possibly owing to the concentration of toxicants in milk.[27] Other dietary associations generally support a decreased risk of PD in those eating healthy diets higher in fruits, vegetables, and grains.[28] Physical activity has been associated with a lower risk of PD, especially in men and particularly at higher intensities of physical activity, although even modest levels reduce risk[29] (**Fig. 1**). The combined

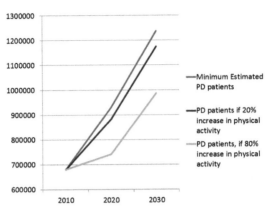

Fig. 1. Estimated number of people with PD in the United States (*blue line*) and the projected reduction in PD if physical activity in adults increases by 20% (*red line*) or 80% (*green line*). Estimates based on Marras and colleagues.[5]

effects of these lifestyle factors seem to be additive, suggesting an approach to disease prevention.[30]

GENETICS AND PATHOPHYSIOLOGY

Specific genetic factors that play a major role in PD risk can be identified in a subset of patients with PD (**Fig. 2**). Polymeropoulos and colleagues[31] identified a mutation in the alpha-synuclein gene, SNCA, in association with rare families with autosomal dominant PD in 1997. Families with these high-penetrant mutations are quite rare, but

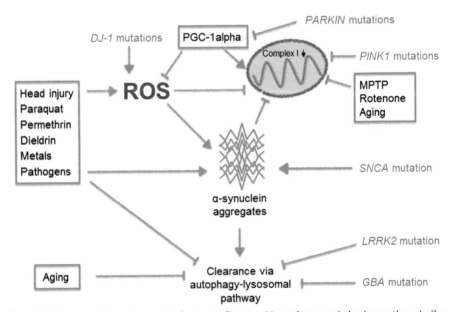

Fig. 2. Environmental and genetic factors influence PD pathogenesis by impacting similar pathways, including mitochondrial function, oxidative stress, alpha-synuclein aggregation, and clearance pathways for abnormal proteins.

this seminal discovery led to the recognition that alpha-synuclein comprises a major component of Lewy bodies even in sporadic patients with PD. The later discovery of autosomal-dominant PD families with alpha-synuclein gene duplications or triplications added to other data indicating that high levels of alpha-synuclein contribute to the pathogenesis of PD.[32]

Mutations in the PARKIN[33] and PINK1[34] genes are causes of early onset autosomal-recessive PD. Both PARKIN and PINK1 have been linked to a cellular pathway involving the preferential degradation in lysosomes of dysfunctional mitochondria through macroautophagy, a process termed "mitophagy." Loss of function of these genes leads to impaired mitophagy, resulting in the accumulation of dysfunctional mitochondria. PARKIN also indirectly regulates levels of an important transcriptional regulator, PGC-1alpha, which coordinately regulates the expression of genes required for mitochondrial biogenesis as well as multiple antioxidant defenses.[35] PGC-1alpha levels also are low in sporadic PD,[36] suggesting that these data are relevant beyond rare genetic forms of PD. These genetic links to both mitochondrial degradation and to mitochondrial biogenesis implicate dysfunction of mitochondrial turnover in PD.

These genetic data are complemented by many other lines of data implicating mitochondrial dysfunction in the pathogenesis of PD. For example, exposure to a toxin, 1-methyl-4-phenyl-1,2,3,6-tetrahydropyridine, causes a rapid onset parkinsonian phenotype and death of dopaminergic neurons in the SN, likely owing to inhibition of mitochondrial complex I activity. Chronic exposure of rodents to rotenone, also a potent mitochondrial complex I inhibitor, also causes preferential degeneration of dopaminergic neurons,[37] and exposure to pesticides (including rotenone) is a risk factor for PD.[38]

Mutations in the DJ-1 gene also cause autosomal-recessive early onset PD.[39] DJ-1 has antioxidant effects through multiple mechanisms, including regulation of NRF2, a transcription factor the upregulates multiple antioxidant defenses, and by stimulating glutathione synthesis.[40]

Mutations in the *LRRK2* gene are associated with autosomal-dominant PD with incomplete penetrance (about 25% for the G2019S mutation, but much higher for the R144G mutation), and are present in about 1% to 2% of all patients with PD and 5% in familial PD, but higher in some populations such as patients of Ashkenazi Jewish ancestry and in North African Berbers.[41] Prior studies suggest that mutations in LRRK2 lead to increased kinase activity,[42] and that LRRK2 kinase inhibitors may be protective,[43] although the possibility of a role for loss of LRRK2 function has been raised.[44]

Another common genetic factor contributing to PD risk relates to mutations in the GBA gene associated with autosomal recessive Gaucher's disease.[45] Carriers of a GBA mutation have an approximately 4-fold increased risk of PD, although the risk varies with different GBA mutations. Some studies suggest an increased risk of dementia in GBA mutation associated PD.[46] PD-linked GBA mutations cause a loss of activity of the lysosomal enzyme glucocerebrosidase (GCase), and agents that upregulate GCase activity and an agent targeting "substrate reduction" have shown promise in animal models and are now moving forward in clinical trials.[47]

Neuroinflammation previously was often viewed only as a response to ongoing neurodegeneration. More recent studies suggest that neuroinflammation might be a significant and essential upstream contributor to alpha-synuclein aggregation and to the neurodegenerative process,[48] and epidemiologic studies have provided evidence of associations between diseases with peripheral inflammation (eg, type 2 diabetes and inflammatory bowel disease) and elevated PD risk.[49,50] Genetic studies also have linked HLA gene variants with the risk of late-onset PD.[51]

PD genetics are complex. Common variants may contribute to PD risk, and can interact with other genetic factors and with environmental factors. The most recent large genome-wide association study identified 70 loci that affect PD risk.[52] Several of these loci are close to genes involved in the lysosomal-autophagy system and in immunity, which are both functions expected to play important roles in the handling of misfolded alpha-synuclein. Acquired (somatic) mitochondrial DNA mutations are increased in SN neurons in early PD and also may play a role.[53] Epigenetic factors also may contribute to PD pathogenesis.[54]

Given the strong genetic and experimental data linking alpha-synuclein toxicity to PD, many potential neuroprotective strategies have focused on mechanisms for clearing away alpha-synuclein aggregates.[55,56] Clinical studies currently are underway using infusion of monoclonal antibodies to target oligomeric alpha-synuclein, or using an active vaccine strategy. Other strategies use more indirect approaches, such as ongoing studies of nilotinib, a c-abl inhibitor, that may decrease inflammation and promote clearance of alpha-synuclein.[57] Additional strategies that specifically target genetically defined subpopulations, such as LRRK2 kinase inhibitors or GCase activators, are moving forward in clinical trials. Although currently genetic testing has a limited role clinically, already it is an important research tool, and one can envision a not-too-distant future when genetic testing will be routine for all patients with PD to guide the selection of targeted therapies.

ALPHA-SYNUCLEIN AGGREGATION AND SPREAD OF PATHOLOGY
Alpha-Synuclein Aggregation

The presence of Lewy pathology is pathognomonic for sporadic PD, although some rare inherited genetic forms of PD that exhibit loss of SN dopaminergic neurons do not display these protein aggregates.[58] Alpha-synuclein is normally enriched in synapses where it is thought to participate in synaptic vesicle function.[59] Alpha-synuclein is also present in non-neuronal cells, for example, liver, muscle, lymphocytes, and red blood cells,[59] and its normal functional roles are not fully elucidated. In a series of seminal studies, Braak and colleagues[60] proposed that there are 6 stages of Lewy pathology in PD. They suggested that in the first stages the Lewy pathology is limited to the dorsal motor nucleus of the vagal nerve, located on the medulla oblongata and the origin of the nerve fibers innervating the gut and other visceral organs, and the olfactory bulb and closely associated olfactory nucleus. They also suggested that the pathology subsequently spreads in a stereotypic fashion along neural pathways throughout the brain, not reaching the SN until the third neuropathologic stage, and eventually involving the cerebral hemispheres in the terminal sixth stage.[60] The Braak staging model is based on post mortem observations, and it has not been possible to obtain definitive proof that pathology spreads in accordance with the Braak stages.[61] Indeed, some subsequent reports indicate that the anatomic pattern of Lewy pathology in some people clinically diagnosed with PD is not consistent with the Braak staging.[62] Still, this model has gained significant traction over the past 2 decades, and it has been proposed that the earliest stages of Lewy pathology (before the SN is engaged) are coupled to the symptoms and signs of premotor PD (discussed elsewhere int his article).[63] Notably, alpha-synuclein aggregates have been reported in the gut of neurologically normal people[64] and around 10% of people who die without a diagnosis of PD still display alpha-synuclein aggregates in the brain (so-called incidental Lewy Body disease) and show mild levels of SN dopaminergic neuronal loss.[65] These observations suggest that these people had elevated risk of developing PD or a related synucleinopathy if they had lived longer.

Table 1
Partial list of key genetic factors associated with PD

Gene	Gene Product	Inheritance	Mutation Types	Penetrance	Age of Onset	Frequency	Notes
SNCA	Alpha-synuclein	AD	Point mutations; duplications; triplications	High	Late (earlier onset with triplications)	Very rare	Earlier onset for triplications compared with duplications
PRKN	Parkin	AR	Multiple, including point mutations; deletions, duplication, (loss of function)	High	Early, often teens or 20s	Rare, 3%–7% with onset 30–45; ≤50% with onset <25	Role in protein degradation; mitophagy
PINK1	PINK1	AR	–	High	Early	Rare (2%–4% of early onset cases)	Role in mitophagy
LRRK2	Leucine rich repeat kinase 2	AD	G2019S; many other point mutations	Moderate (~25%)	Late	~1%–2% of all PD cases; higher in Ashkenazi Jews, North African Berbers, and Basques	Mutations cause increased kinase activity
DJ-1	DJ-1	AR	Point mutations	High	Early	Rare (1% of early onset cases)	Protects against oxidative stress
GBA	Glucocerebrosidase	Mixed	Point mutations (loss of function)	Low (~4-fold increased risk)	Late	5%–10% of all patients with PD; higher in Ashkenazi Jews	Lysosomal enzyme

Abbreviations: AD, autosomal dominant; AR, autosomal recessive; SNCA, alpha-synuclein gene.

See the following works for more comprehensive reviews: Schulte C, Gasser T. Genetic basis of Parkinson's disease: inheritance, penetrance, and expression. Appl Clin Genet. 2011;4:67–80; and Lin MK, Farrer MJ. Genetics and genomics of Parkinson's disease. Genome Med. 2014;6(6):48.

A Prion-Like Role for Alpha-Synuclein Assemblies?

Different alpha-synuclein assemblies have been shown to be secreted by neurons, via a process that is elevated if the lysosomal-autophagy system is inhibited, and then be taken up by neighboring neurons where they are capable of seeding monomeric alpha-synuclein into Lewy-like aggregates.[66] The realization that misfolded alpha-synuclein exhibit such prion-like properties has increased the spotlight on the Braak staging system. Because these pathogenic alpha-synuclein assemblies can be transported intra-axonally to interconnected nuclei, prion-like behavior of alpha-synuclein assemblies might explain how Lewy pathology propagates from one brain region to another[66] and could be consistent with the spread of alpha-synuclein pathology proposed by Braak and colleagues.

An important question is what might be the initial trigger of alpha-synuclein aggregation. One model proposes that numerous factors are involved, including some of the environmental risk factors we discussed earlier, that is, pesticides and environmental pollutants, as well as common pathogens (eg, viruses, bacteria and fungi) that all can gain access to alpha-synuclein containing cells initially in the olfactory system and gut.[67] For the most part, these aggregates are handled by normal cellular proteostatic mechanisms and do not lead to spreading Lewy pathology. In the simultaneous presence of facilitating factors, for example, aging, genetic predisposition, and peripheral inflammation, the model proposes that alpha-synuclein aggregates can bypass normal clearance and cause synucleinopathy in the brain.[67] Although a role for alpha-synuclein is well-established in PD, it is worth noting that it remains controversial whether or not the aggregates themselves are pathogenic[68] (**Table 1**).

SUMMARY

PD is a complex disorder, with both environmental and genetic factors converging on a common set of pathways including mitochondrial dysfunction, oxidative stress, protein aggregation, impaired autophagy and neuroinflammation. Decreasing the burden of PD can be approached with a 2-pronged strategy: the implementation of interventions to reduce modifiable factors such as behavioral or environmental risk factors and the development of drugs targeting the mechanisms of genes or environmental exposures associated with PD. PD incidence is increased in persons with prodromal symptoms such as impaired olfaction, sleep disorders and constipation.[69] Targeting people in this prodromal stage of disease may be an effective strategy for reducing the burden of PD in future decades. Clinical testing of interventions aimed at identifying disease-modifying therapies thus far has yielded mainly negative results, perhaps in part because the pathophysiological factors contributing to PD differ between patients. The lack of clinically proven success at slowing disease progression highlights the need for more research to better understand the molecular pathophysiology of subtypes of PD.

REFERENCES

1. Parkinson J. An essay on the shaking palsy. London: Sherwood, Neely, and Jones; 1817.
2. Sung VW, Nicholas AP. Nonmotor symptoms in Parkinson's disease: expanding the view of Parkinson's disease beyond a pure motor, pure dopaminergic problem. Neurol Clin 2013;31(3 Suppl):S1–16.
3. Poewe W, Seppi K, Tanner CM, et al. Parkinson disease. Nat Rev Dis Primers 2017;3:17013.

4. Fearnley JM, Lees AJ. Ageing and Parkinson's disease: substantia nigra regional selectivity. Brain 1991;114(Pt 5):2283–301.
5. Marras C, Beck JC, Bower JH, et al. Prevalence of Parkinson's disease across North America. NPJ Parkinsons Dis 2018;4:21.
6. Twelves D, Perkins KS, Counsell C. Systematic review of incidence studies of Parkinson's disease. Mov Disord 2003;18(1):19–31.
7. Pinter B, Diem-Zangerl A, Wenning GK, et al. Mortality in Parkinson's disease: a 38-year follow-up study. Mov Disord 2015;30(2):266–9.
8. Dorsey ER, Sherer T, Okun MS, et al. The emerging evidence of the Parkinson pandemic. J Parkinsons Dis 2018;8(s1):S3–8.
9. Kaltenboeck A, Johnson SJ, Davis MR, et al. Direct costs and survival of medicare beneficiaries with early and advanced Parkinson's disease. Parkinsonism Relat Disord 2012;18(4):321–6.
10. Goldman SM, Marek K, Ottman R, et al. Concordance for Parkinson's disease in twins: a 20-year update. Ann Neurol 2019;85(4):600–5.
11. Tanner CM, Goldman SM, Ross GW, et al. The disease intersection of susceptibility and exposure: chemical exposures and neurodegenerative disease risk. Alzheimers Dement 2014;10(3 Suppl):S213–25.
12. Goldman SM. Environmental toxins and Parkinson's disease. Annu Rev Pharmacol Toxicol 2014;54:141–64.
13. Furlong M, Tanner CM, Goldman SM, et al. Protective glove use and hygiene habits modify the associations of specific pesticides with Parkinson's disease. Environ Int 2015;75:144–50.
14. Kamel F, Goldman SM, Umbach DM, et al. Dietary fat intake, pesticide use, and Parkinson's disease. Parkinsonism Relat Disord 2014;20(1):82–7.
15. Weisskopf MG, Knekt P, O'Reilly EJ, et al. Polychlorinated biphenyls in prospectively collected serum and Parkinson's disease risk. Mov Disord 2012;27(13):1659–65.
16. Goldman SM, Quinlan PJ, Ross GW, et al. Solvent exposures and Parkinson disease risk in twins. Ann Neurol 2012;71(6):776–84.
17. Criswell SR, Nielsen SS, Warden M, et al. [(18)F]FDOPA positron emission tomography in manganese-exposed workers. Neurotoxicology 2018;64:43–9.
18. Racette BA, Searles Nielsen S, Criswell SR, et al. Dose-dependent progression of parkinsonism in manganese-exposed welders. Neurology 2017;88(4):344–51.
19. Harischandra DS, Rokad D, Neal ML, et al. Manganese promotes the aggregation and prion-like cell-to-cell exosomal transmission of alpha-synuclein. Sci Signal 2019;12(572) [pii:eaau4543].
20. Kenborg L, Lassen CF, Hansen J, et al. Parkinson's disease and other neurodegenerative disorders among welders: a Danish cohort study. Mov Disord 2012;27(10):1283–9.
21. Finkelstein MM, Jerrett M. A study of the relationships between Parkinson's disease and markers of traffic-derived and environmental manganese air pollution in two Canadian cities. Environ Res 2007;104(3):420–32.
22. Kenborg L, Rugbjerg K, Lee PC, et al. Head injury and risk for Parkinson disease: results from a Danish case-control study. Neurology 2015;84(11):1098–103.
23. Morens DM, Davis JW, Grandinetti A, et al. Epidemiologic observations on Parkinson's disease: incidence and mortality in a prospective study of middle-aged men. Neurology 1996;46(4):1044–50.
24. Ritz B, Ascherio A, Checkoway H, et al. Pooled analysis of tobacco use and risk of Parkinson disease. Arch Neurol 2007;64(7):990–7.

25. Ross GW, Abbott RD, Petrovitch H, et al. Association of coffee and caffeine intake with the risk of Parkinson disease. JAMA 2000;283(20):2674–9.

26. Ascherio A, Schwarzschild MA. The epidemiology of Parkinson's disease: risk factors and prevention. Lancet Neurol 2016;15(12):1257–72.

27. Park M, Ross GW, Petrovitch H, et al. Consumption of milk and calcium in midlife and the future risk of Parkinson disease. Neurology 2005;64(6):1047–51.

28. Gao X, Chen H, Fung TT, et al. Prospective study of dietary pattern and risk of Parkinson disease. Am J Clin Nutr 2007;86(5):1486–94.

29. Yang F, Trolle Lagerros Y, Bellocco R, et al. Physical activity and risk of Parkinson's disease in the Swedish National March cohort. Brain 2015;138(Pt 2): 269–75.

30. Kim IY, O'Reilly EJ, Hughes KC, et al. Integration of risk factors for Parkinson disease in 2 large longitudinal cohorts. Neurology 2018;90(19):e1646–53.

31. Polymeropoulos MH, Lavedan C, Leroy E, et al. Mutation in the alpha-synuclein gene identified in families with Parkinson's disease. Science 1997;276(5321): 2045–7.

32. Singleton AB, Farrer M, Johnson J, et al. alpha-Synuclein locus triplication causes Parkinson's disease. Science 2003;302:841.

33. Kitada T, Asakawa S, Hattori N, et al. Mutations in the parkin gene cause autosomal recessive juvenile parkinsonism. Nature 1998;392(6676):605–8.

34. Valente EM, Abou-Sleiman PM, Caputo V, et al. Hereditary early-onset Parkinson's disease caused by mutations in PINK1. Science 2004;304(5674):1158–60.

35. Shin JH, Ko HS, Kang H, et al. PARIS (ZNF746) repression of PGC-1alpha contributes to neurodegeneration in Parkinson's disease. Cell 2011;144(5):689–702.

36. Zheng B, Liao Z, Locascio JJ, et al. PGC-1alpha, a potential therapeutic target for early intervention in Parkinson's disease. Sci Transl Med 2010;2(52):52ra73.

37. Greenamyre JT, Betarbet R, Sherer TB. The rotenone model of Parkinson's disease: genes, environment and mitochondria. Parkinsonism Relat Disord 2003; 9(Suppl 2):S59–64.

38. Tanner CM, Kamel F, Ross GW, et al. Rotenone, paraquat, and Parkinson's disease. Environ Health Perspect 2011;119(6):866–72.

39. Bonifati V, Rizzu P, van Baren MJ, et al. Mutations in the DJ-1 gene associated with autosomal recessive early-onset parkinsonism. Science 2003;299(5604): 256–9.

40. Raninga PV, Di Trapani G, Tonissen KF. The multifaceted roles of DJ-1 as an antioxidant. Adv Exp Med Biol 2017;1037:67–87.

41. Alessi DR, Sammler E. LRRK2 kinase in Parkinson's disease. Science 2018; 360(6384):36–7.

42. West AB, Moore DJ, Choi C, et al. Parkinson's disease-associated mutations in LRRK2 link enhanced GTP-binding and kinase activities to neuronal toxicity. Hum Mol Genet 2007;16(2):223–32.

43. Hatcher JM, Choi HG, Alessi DR, et al. Small-molecule inhibitors of LRRK2. Adv Neurobiol 2017;14:241–64.

44. Giaime E, Tong Y, Wagner LK, et al. Age-dependent dopaminergic neurodegeneration and impairment of the autophagy-lysosomal pathway in LRRK-deficient mice. Neuron 2017;96(4):796–807.e6.

45. Clark LN, Nicolai A, Afridi S, et al. Pilot association study of the beta-glucocerebrosidase N370S allele and Parkinson's disease in subjects of Jewish ethnicity. Mov Disord 2005;20(1):100–3.

46. Riboldi GM, Di Fonzo AB. GBA, Gaucher disease, and Parkinson's disease: from genetic to clinic to new therapeutic approaches. Cells 2019;8(4) [pii:E364].

47. Balestrino R, Schapira AHV. Glucocerebrosidase and Parkinson disease: molecular, clinical, and therapeutic implications. Neuroscientist 2018;24(5):540–59.
48. Kannarkat GT, Boss JM, Tansey MG. The role of innate and adaptive immunity in Parkinson's disease. J Parkinsons Dis 2013;3(4):493–514.
49. Rolli-Derkinderen M, Leclair-Visonneau L, Bourreille A, et al. Is Parkinson's disease a chronic low-grade inflammatory bowel disease? J Neurol 2019. https://doi.org/10.1007/s00415-019-09321-0.
50. De Pablo-Fernandez E, Goldacre R, Pakpoor J, et al. Association between diabetes and subsequent Parkinson disease: a record-linkage cohort study. Neurology 2018;91(2):e139–42.
51. Hamza TH, Zabetian CP, Tenesa A, et al. Common genetic variation in the HLA region is associated with late-onset sporadic Parkinson's disease. Nat Genet 2010;42(9):781–5.
52. Nalls MA, Blauwendraat C, Vallerga CL, et al. Parkinson's disease genetics: identifying novel risk loci, providing causal insights and improving estimates of heritable risk. bioRxiv 2019;388165.
53. Lin MT, Cantuti-Castelvetri I, Zheng K, et al. Somatic mitochondrial DNA mutations in early Parkinson and incidental Lewy body disease. Ann Neurol 2012;71(6):850–4.
54. van Heesbeen HJ, Smidt MP. Entanglement of genetics and epigenetics in Parkinson's disease. Front Neurosci 2019;13:277.
55. Kalia LV, Kalia SK, Lang AE. Disease-modifying strategies for Parkinson's disease. Mov Disord 2015;30(11):1442–50.
56. Savitt D, Jankovic J. Targeting alpha-synuclein in Parkinson's disease: progress towards the development of disease-modifying therapeutics. Drugs 2019;79(8):797–810.
57. Wyse RK, Brundin P, Sherer TB. Nilotinib - differentiating the hope from the hype. J Parkinsons Dis 2016;6(3):519–22.
58. Schneider SA, Alcalay RN. Neuropathology of genetic synucleinopathies with parkinsonism: review of the literature. Mov Disord 2017;32(11):1504–23.
59. Burre J, Sharma M, Sudhof TC. Cell biology and pathophysiology of alpha-synuclein. Cold Spring Harb Perspect Med 2018;8(3).
60. Braak H, Del Tredici K, Rub U, et al. Staging of brain pathology related to sporadic Parkinson's disease. Neurobiol Aging 2003;24(2):197–211.
61. Braak H, Del Tredici K. Neuropathological staging of brain pathology in sporadic Parkinson's disease: separating the wheat from the chaff. J Parkinsons Dis 2017;7(s1):S71–85.
62. Beach TG, Adler CH, Lue L, et al. Unified staging system for Lewy body disorders: correlation with nigrostriatal degeneration, cognitive impairment and motor dysfunction. Acta Neuropathol 2009;117(6):613–34.
63. Postuma RB, Berg D. Advances in markers of prodromal Parkinson disease. Nat Rev Neurol 2016;12(11):622–34.
64. Lionnet A, Leclair-Visonneau L, Neunlist M, et al. Does Parkinson's disease start in the gut? Acta Neuropathol 2018;135(1):1–12.
65. van de Berg WD, Hepp DH, Dijkstra AA, et al. Patterns of alpha-synuclein pathology in incidental cases and clinical subtypes of Parkinson's disease. Parkinsonism Relat Disord 2012;18(Suppl 1):S28–30.
66. Brundin P, Melki R. Prying into the prion hypothesis for Parkinson's disease. J Neurosci 2017;37(41):9808–18.
67. Johnson ME, Stecher B, Labrie V, et al. Triggers, facilitators, and aggravators: redefining Parkinson's disease pathogenesis. Trends Neurosci 2019;42(1):4–13.

68. Espay AJ, Vizcarra JA, Marsili L, et al. Revisiting protein aggregation as pathogenic in sporadic Parkinson and Alzheimer diseases. Neurology 2019;92(7): 329–37.
69. Ross GW, Abbott RD, Petrovitch H, et al. Pre-motor features of Parkinson's disease: the Honolulu-Asia aging study experience. Parkinsonism Relat Disord 2012;18(Suppl 1):S199–202.

Diagnosis and Differential Diagnosis of Parkinson Disease

Stefano Caproni, MD, PhD, Carlo Colosimo, MD, FEAN*

KEYWORDS

- Dementia with Lewy bodies • Parkinsonism • Parkinson disease
- Multiple system atrophy • Progressive supranuclear palsy

KEY POINTS

- In contrast to the common opinion that diagnosing Parkinson disease (PD) is straightforward, several clinicopathological studies found that approximately one-fourth of patients diagnosed as PD during life have an alternative diagnosis (ie, atypical parkinsonism, Alzheimer-type pathology, or vascular encephalopathy) at postmortem.
- In the past 3 decades, a number of criteria and guidelines have been introduced to optimize the diagnosis of PD. As a result of these criteria, the diagnostic accuracy rose from 75% to 82%, but many patients still require the opinion of a movement disorders specialist for the purpose of establishing the diagnosis.
- In determining whether a patient with parkinsonian features has PD or a related disorder, it is important to be aware of "red flags," which are features from the history and examination not expected with PD that suggest another cause of that clinical picture, typically known as parkinsonism.

INTRODUCTION

Parkinson disease (PD) is a common neurodegenerative disorder of the aging population, and its diagnosis is based mainly on clinical features. In contrast to the common opinion that diagnosing PD is straightforward, several clinicopathological studies found that approximately one-fourth of patients diagnosed as PD during life has an alternative diagnosis (ie, atypical parkinsonism, Alzheimer-type pathology, or vascular encephalopathy) at postmortem.[1] In particular, this is true for the initial diagnosis, because the diagnostic accuracy improves during follow-up, achieving the highest positive predictive value in the last evaluations before death.[2] In the past 3 decades, a number of criteria and guidelines have been introduced to optimize the diagnosis of PD. As a result of these criteria, the diagnostic accuracy rose from 75% to 82%, but

Neurology Division, Neuroscience Department, "S. Maria" University Hospital, via Tristano di Joannuccio, Terni 05100, Italy
* Corresponding author.
E-mail address: c.colosimo@aospterni.it

Clin Geriatr Med 36 (2020) 13–24
https://doi.org/10.1016/j.cger.2019.09.014
0749-0690/20/© 2019 Elsevier Inc. All rights reserved.

many patients still require the opinion of a movement disorders specialist for the purpose of establishing the diagnosis.[1]

A task force from a collaborative European Federation of Neurological Societies/Movement Disorders Society-European Section effort produced extensive therapeutic[3,4] and then diagnostic[5] guidelines for PD. The members of this task force highlighted the best clinical and laboratory clues for identification of PD, giving specific recommendations to improve the clinical diagnosis, which had previously been mainly based on the UK Parkinson's Disease Society Brain Bank clinical diagnostic criteria.[6] In addition to these guidelines, the American Academy of Neurology previously published guidelines on the diagnosis of PD and most recently, the International Parkinson's Disease and Movement Disorders Society produced new guidelines based on novel findings of the nonmotor profile of disease, the recognition of PD as a synucleinopathy, identification of genetic causes, novel hypotheses about spread of disease.[7]

In determining whether a patient with parkinsonian features has PD or a related disorder, it is important to be aware of "red flags," which are features from the history and examination not expected with PD that suggest another cause of that clinical picture, typically known as parkinsonism.

Parkinsonism is a general term that refers to a group of movement disorders similar to PD; under this category, there are a number of disorders, some of which have yet to be clearly defined or named. In the early disease process, it is often hard to know whether a person has PD or a condition that mimics it.

Initially proposed by Quinn[8] in 1989 to denote the clinical features that suggested multiple system atrophy (MSA), an increasing number of red flags have been reported over the years with some of them gaining acceptance as part of the standard diagnostic criteria for PD, atypical parkinsonian disorders, secondary parkinsonism (above all, drug-induced parkinsonism), or other heredodegenerative diseases[9,10] (**Box 1**).

PARKINSON DISEASE

Bradykinesia is the core feature of PD, exhibiting unilaterally as the other core features. It is defined as slowness of movement associated with decrement in amplitude or speed as movements are continued.[7] At disease onset, it is often misinterpreted by patients as weakness, and has many facets, depending of the affected body part (head, trunk, or limbs), resulting in a variety of clinical signs (**Box 2**).[11]

In addition to bradykinesia, patients with PD present at least 1 other cardinal feature, such as muscular rigidity, rest tremor, and postural instability.[6] Axial or limb rigidity is characterized by an increased resistance to passive movement and usually is manifested by the "cogwheeling" phenomenon. Rest tremor at a frequency of 4 to 6 Hz is usually present in the extremities (involving the thumb and the forefinger in the "pill-rolling" form), in the chin, in the lips, and the tongue. It is worsened by stress and excitement. The main differential diagnosis for parkinsonian tremor is essential tremor (ET), which is a bilateral action tremor that can also involve the head or voice, the latter not typically seen in PD. ET is hereditary in at least half of the cases and can be distinguished from PD tremor clinically and if necessary also by means of laboratory tests, such as DaTSCAN or midbrain sonography, which are normal in ET.[12] A detailed description of tremor is the objective of Stephen G. Reich's article, "Does This Patient Have Parkinson's Disease or Essential Tremor?," elsewhere in this issue.

Postural instability is an impairment of balance, that is, the ability to maintain or change posture such as when standing and walking. It represents one of the most disabling symptoms in the advanced stages of PD, as it is associated with increased falls and loss of independence. With the progression of the disease, patients frequently exhibit a

---

Box 1
Classification of parkinsonian disorders

Idiopathic form
  Parkinson disease (sporadic and familial)

Atypical Degenerative Parkinsonism
  Multiple system atrophy (parkinsonian MSA-P, and cerebellar type MSA-C)
  Progressive supranuclear palsy
  Corticobasal syndrome
  Lewy body dementia

Secondary Parkinsonism
  Dementia Syndromes
    Alzheimer disease
    Frontotemporal dementia
  Lytico-Bodig (Guam parkinsonism-dementia-amyotrophic lateral sclerosis)
  Progressive pallidal atrophy
  Vascular
  Drug-induced
  Hemiatrophy-hemiparkinsonism
  Normal pressure hydrocephalus
  Hypoxia
  Postencephalitic
  Metabolic
  Toxic
  Posttraumatic
  Neoplasm

Heredodegenerative Diseases
  Neurodegeneration with brain iron accumulation
  Huntington disease
  X-Linked dystonia-parkinsonism
  Neuroacanthocytosis
  Wilson disease

Adapted from Colosimo C. The differential diagnosis of Parkinsonism: a clinical approach. In: Colosimo C, Riley DE, Wenning GK, editors. Handbook of atypical Parkinsonism. Cambridge: Cambridge University Press; 2011. p. 126-41; with permission.

---

loss of postural reflexes, in particular when standing up or changing direction while walking. Conversely, when exhibiting in the early stages of a subject diagnosed with PD, it should be considered a "red flag" for the differential diagnosis. Postural instability can be clinically evaluated by pull test, in which the physician stands behind the patient and briskly pulls him or her backward by the shoulders. This test is considered positive if the patient takes more than 2 steps to regain balance, or if the patient falls if unsupported by the examiner. In addition, with the disease progression, disability is worsened by the appearance a flexed body posture, which usually begins in the arms and spreads to involve the legs and the entire body. Extreme flexion of the trunk is called camptocormia, whereas severe lateral tilting of the trunk is referred to as Pisa syndrome; they can sometimes be observed in combination. These features usually present in advanced stages of PD, whereas if observed in the early stages may be considered as "red flags" for an atypical parkinsonian syndrome.[13,14]

Another cardinal motor sign that can be observed in the middle or advanced stage of the disease is the freezing phenomenon, a transient inability to perform active movement (also known as motor block). It usually affects the legs (freezing of gait), but can also involve eyelid opening or closing, writing, or speaking. It is much less frequent when the patient is going up or down steps than when walking on level

---

Box 2
Clinical features of bradykinesia in different body parts

Head
  Hypomimia
  Hypometric saccades
  Impaired upward gaze and convergence
  Glabellar tap sign (Meyerson sign)
  Hypophonia
  Sialorrhea

Trunk
  Slowness in initiating movement on command
  Impaired arising from a chair and turning on bed
  Impaired shoulder shrugging

Upper Limb
  Slowness in daily activities
  Reduced spontaneous movement
  Decrement amplitude with repetitive movements
  Micrographia
  Decreased arm swing when walking

Lower Limb
  Short and slow steps when walking
  Shuffling walk
  Decrement amplitude with repetitive movements

Adapted from Fahn S, Kang UJ. Parkinson disease. In: Louis ED, Mayer SA, Lewys P, editors. Merrit's neurology. 13th ed. Philadelphia: Wolters Kluwer; 2016. p. 704-21; with permission.

---

ground, and can be overcome by visual clues. The combination of loss of postural reflexes and freezing of gait dramatically contributes to a higher risk of falls.[15]

The clinical impact of the previously mentioned cardinal signs of PD vary significantly with reference to their impact on activities of daily living. A detailed and standardized scoring of individual motor (and nonmotor) signs and symptoms of PD can be assessed by the Unified Parkinson's Disease Rating Scale (UPDRS), and its updated version from the Movement Disorder Society (MDS-UPDRS).[16–19] The progression of the motor features of PD, from unilateral to bilateral (stage 1 to stage 2) to the loss of postural reflexes (stage 3 and 4) to becoming wheelchair bound (stage 5) is captured by the Hoehn and Yahr clinical staging scale (**Table 1**).[16] It is important to note though that although PD is progressive, the rate and severity of progression is highly variable and not all patients progress through all of the Hoehn and Yahr stages.

In addition to its cardinal motor features, PD is also characterized by nonmotor symptoms that aid in the diagnosis and several are included in the diagnostic criteria.[7] These nonmotor features of PD are present throughout the evolution of the disease, and some of them, such as hyposmia, depression, constipation, and dream enactment (eg, REM sleep behavior disorder [RBD]) often develop in the prodromal stage of PD, up to 5 to 10 years before the presentation of motor symptoms.[20,21]

Other nonmotor symptoms of PD,[22] like sensory features (pain, akathisia, and restless legs syndrome) can also precede or appear simultaneously with motor features and may respond to dopaminergic treatment.[23] With progression of the disease, a significant number of patients with PD develop autonomic disturbances, such as urinary incontinence, sexual dysfunction, orthostatic hypotension, and constipation, that critically worsen quality of life, often more than the motor symptoms of PD; some autonomic symptoms (such as orthostatic hypotension) may also increase the risk of

Table 1	
Modified Hoehn and Yahr staging scale for Parkinson disease	
Stage 0	No sign of disease
Stage 1	Unilateral features
Stage 1.5	Unilateral plus midline/axial involvement
Stage 2	Bilateral features, without impairment of balance
Stage 2.5	Mild bilateral disease, with an abnormal pull test but with falling avoidance
Stage 3	Mild to moderate bilateral disease; minor postural instability, but physically independent
Stage 4	Severe disability; necessary of supervision to avoid falling
Stage 5	Wheelchair bound or bedridden

Adapted from Fahn S, Elton RL, UPDRS Program Members. Unified Parkinson's disease rating scale. In: Fahn S, Marsden CD, Goldstein M, Calne DB, editors. Recent developments in Parkinson's disease, Vol. 2. Florham Park, NJ: Macmillan Healthcare Information; 1987. p. 153-163; 293-304; with permission.

falls, further reducing independence.[24] Neuropsychiatric symptoms are predominantly observed in the mid or late stages of PD and represent some of the disabling features for patients as well as significant challenges for clinicians. Anxiety and depression are very common in PD; additional neuropsychiatric features include reduced attention span, visuospatial impairment, and apathy associated with increased dependence on the caregiver. Mild cognitive dysfunction in PD often proceeds to overt dementia, which may be accompanied by hallucinations and delusions. Several of the medications used to treat PD, particularly the dopamine agonists, causes impulse control disorder,[20,25] such as pathologic gambling, sexuality, and shopping, among others (**Box 3**).

In conclusion, the diagnosis of PD hinges on recognizing a typical form, with unilateral onset, characterized by bradykinesia, rest tremor, and cogwheel rigidity, responding to levodopa. Clinicians should consider "red flags," which are features not expected with PD and suggest an alternative diagnosis, usually a parkinsonian syndrome.

Although the most common cause of parkinsonism is PD, the differential diagnosis includes many other causes of parkinsonism. Aside from drug-induced parkinsonism, related to drug-induced changes in the basal ganglia motor circuit secondary to dopaminergic receptor blockade, the most common mimickers of PD are parkinsonian syndromes, such as MSA and progressive supranuclear palsy. These "cousins" of PD are distinguished by first recognizing that the patient with parkinsonism has features not expected with PD (such as bilateral onset of motor features, absence of rest tremor, severe bulbar symptoms, early falls or dementia, or a poor response to levodopa), as well as recognizing the characteristic features of specific parkinsonian syndromes, to be discussed as follows.

MULTIPLE SYSTEM ATROPHY

MSA is a sporadic neurodegenerative disease clinically characterized by 2 main motor features, parkinsonism or cerebellar ataxia combined with dysautonomia. These motor features are the basis for classifying forms with predominant parkinsonism (MSA-P), that is the most common phenotype in Europe and America, or cerebellar features (MSA-C), predominant in East Asia. The typical presentation of MSA is parkinsonism that is poorly responsive to levodopa. The term MSA incorporates what was

---

Box 3
Nonmotor features of Parkinson disease

Sensory symptoms
  Hyposmia
  Paresthesias
  Pain
  Akathisia
  Restless legs syndrome
  Fatigue

Autonomic symptoms
  Constipation
  Orthostatic hypotension
  Incontinence
  Sexual dysfunctions
  Sweating (excessive or diminished)
  Reduced gastric emptying

Neuropsychiatric symptoms
  Anxiety
  Depression
  Apathy
  Dependence by caregiver
  Mild cognitive impairment
  Dementia
  Hallucinations
  Psychosis
  Compulsive behaviors

Sleep disturbances
  Sleep fragmentation
  Excessive daytime sleepiness
  Rapid eye movement sleep behavior disorder

---

previously termed Shy-Drager syndrome, striatonigral degeneration and olivoponto-cerebellar atrophy recognizing that clinically and pathologically these are all varieties of MSA.[8] Beyond motor features, MSA may also present with a variety of autonomic, pyramidal, cognitive, and behavioral symptoms, highlighting the peculiar multisystemic nature of the disease[26] and the challenge of making an early diagnosis.

Unlike the tremor associated with PD, the tremor observed in two-thirds of the patients with MSA is of the postural and kinetic type, and can be accompanied by touch-sensitive and stimulus-sensitive myoclonus.[10] Patients with MSA, in particular MSA-P type, commonly exhibit more pronounced bradykinesia than patients with PD, with a relative symmetry and a poor response to levodopa, even if up to one-third of patients show an initial improvement with pharmacologic treatment.[27,28] This initial improvement observed in some patients with MSA-P is practically never as dramatic as seen with PD, is usually not long-lasting, and is usually not associated with levodopa-induced fluctuations and dyskinesia seen eventually in most patients with PD. In patients with MSA, rigidity may be accompanied by spasticity, and balance difficulty is pronounced and often appears early, although is not usually associated with recurrent falls.[29] The facial appearance of patients with MSA is sometimes characterized by atypical dystonia or dyskinesia, which mainly affects the orofacial muscles and occasionally resembles "risus sardonicus" observed in Wilson disease.[30]

In contrast to PD, patients with MSA have preserved olfactory function.[10] Sleep disturbances, including RBD, are more common in MSA than in PD, and patients with

MSA may have nocturnal inspiratory stridor and obstructive sleep apnea that can cause sudden death.[31]

Among nonmotor symptoms, autonomic failure is part of the diagnostic criteria of MSA, and includes early orthostatic hypotension, constipation, early and often prominent dysphagia, early urinary incontinence, and erectile dysfunction.[10] With regard to neuropsychiatric disturbances, patients with MSA usually exhibit executive dysfunction and pseudobulbar crying or laughing spells, with only a minority of cases progressing to full-blown dementia.[10]

Among the aforementioned clinical features, it is important to underline the main "red flags" that can help to distinguish PD from MSA. These include rapid clinical deterioration, such as progressing to use of a wheelchair within 3 years of onset of symptoms ("wheelchair sign"), early postural instability, abnormal postures (Pisa syndrome, antecollis (neck flexion), and contractures of hand or feet), bulbar dysfunction (early dysphonia, dysarthria, and dysphagia), early autonomic failure, respiratory dysfunction, and emotional incontinence.[26]

Laboratory investigations may help to distinguish the various forms of parkinsonism. DaTSCAN, which is a marker of nigrostriatal degeneration, is abnormal in both PD and MSA (and most other parkinsonian syndromes), and as such is not useful to make this distinction. MRI, which is normal in PD, can show specific abnormalities in MSA, such as the "hot cross bun" sign (a cross hyperintensity of the pons, due to its atrophy) and bilateral putaminal hyperintensity. However, these changes do not usual appear early in the disease, limiting therefore their practical value, emphasizing the need to look carefully for red flags that cast doubt on the diagnosis of PD.

PROGRESSIVE SUPRANUCLEAR PALSY

Progressive supranuclear palsy (PSP) was first described by Richardson and colleagues[32] as a pre-senile sporadic neurodegenerative disease clinically characterized by a combination of supranuclear vertical ophthalmoplegia (inability to move the eyes up and down), pseudobulbar palsy, nuchal dystonia, and frontolimbic dementia. Successive pathologic studies pointed out that PSP is a tauopathy characterized by hyperphosphorylated tau protein deposition forming neurofibrillary tangles in cerebral neocortex, pallidum, subthalamic nucleus, substantia nigra, periaqueductal gray matter, superior colliculi, and dentate nucleus.[33] The core clinical diagnostic features of PSP have been collected in several sets of criteria, evolving in the past 2 decades, and recently revised by the MDS PSP study group.[34]

Resting tremor is usually absent in PSP, expect for the PSP-parkinsonism (PSP-P) phenotype, that can show a moderate response to levodopa. A symmetric onset and rapid progression are characteristic of bradykinesia in PSP, and unlike PD, in PSP the bradykinesia and rigidity are more axial (neck and trunk) than appendicular (limbs). In occasional cases, PSP can manifest as a pure akinetic syndrome with early freezing of gait.[35] Axial rigidity (with primary extensor neck rigidity and retrocollis [neck extension]) is also characteristic of the classic phenotype of PSP.[33]

Postural instability associated with early backward falls during the first course of disease is a cardinal feature of PSP. Moreover, patients with PSP have difficulty rising from the sitting position; they also tend to sit and turn "en bloc" (tend to raise their feet when sitting and minimally rotate the trunk while turning around). In contrast to PD, patients with PSP ambulate with an erect posture and abducted arms.[36]

With regard to facial appearance, in PSP a peculiar wide-eyed, nonblinking, staring expression is more frequent then simple hypomimia, as observed in PD; this is often referred to as a look of anguish or surprise due to deep facial grooves and contraction of the frontalis. The most distinctive feature of PSP is impairment of vertical saccadic eye movement, eventually leading to vertical ophthalmoplegia. Saccades are the rapid movements that shift gaze; vertical pursuit eye movements are disproportionately preserved in PSP so having the patient follow a finger is not a good test when considering PSP, as it may be normal. Instead, patients should be asked to shift their gaze between targets. Vertical supranuclear palsy initially affects downgaze (upgaze paresis may be also related to aging and, therefore, not specific). The preservation of oculocephalic reflexes is consistent with the supranuclear origin of the disturbance; that is, when the head is moved vertically, they eyes demonstrate a full range of movement (when the head is extended the eyes move down in the orbit and vice versa). These key features are accompanied by reduced blink rate, convergence insufficiency, eyelid apraxia (inability to open the gently closed eye), and compensatory eyebrow elevation.[37]

Among nonmotor symptoms, PSP is not usually characterized by specific olfactory, sleep, sensory, and autonomic disturbances, but is usually associated with profound cognitive difficulties[33] primarily reflecting frontal lobe dysfunction, and PSP may present with cognitive and behavioral impairment.

MRI can help in diagnosing PSP showing significant midbrain atrophy ("Hummingbird sign" in sagittal plane, "Morning Glory sign" in axial plane) (**Fig. 1**). Furthermore, morphometric studies focused on midbrain and superior cerebellar peduncle found that an index calculated with a specific formula ("magnetic resonance parkinsonism index" = area of pons/area of midbrain × medial cerebellar peduncle diameter/superior cerebellar peduncle diameter) can differentiate PSP from PD and MSA.[38]

CORTICOBASAL DEGENERATION

Another tauopathy related to PSP is corticobasal degeneration (CBD). Despite published diagnostic criteria,[39] the clinical diagnosis of CBD is confirmed in only approximately 50% of autopsies and therefore the term CBD is reserved for a pathologically confirmed diagnosis and during life, it is referred to as corticobasal syndrome (CBS).[40]

CBS is clinically characterized by a combination of levodopa-unresponsive parkinsonism with early loss of balance, severe unilateral limb dystonia, and a variety of focal cortical deficits reflecting, as its name implies, a combination of signs referable to the basal ganglia (parkinsonism, rigidity, dystonia) and the cortex (apraxia,

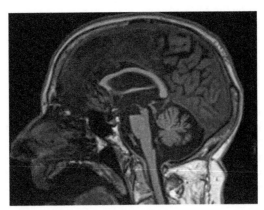

Fig. 1. A 65-year-old male patient suffering from PSP: a sagittal T1-weighted image showing the hummingbird sign (severe mesencephalic atrophy).

agraphesthesia, astereognosis, myoclonus, and aphasia). CBD pathology reveals the presence of enlarged achromatic neurons in parietal and frontal lobes, along with nigral and striatal degeneration, without the occurrence of Lewy bodies.

Resting tremor is only occasionally present in CBS, whereas myoclonic jerks of the limb, which clinically resemble tremor ("jerky tremor"), are common. Typically, rigidity is accompanied by dystonic features and contractures. Rigidity in CBS is associated with marked unilateral motor impairment, due to kinetic and ideomotor apraxia. In some cases, the involuntary movement of a limb (in particular an arm) that floats in the space without the patient's discernment can be observed (alien limb phenomenon).[41] CBS, unlike most other causes of parkinsonism (except PD) usually begins unilaterally, and that is an important diagnostic clue.

In the later stages of CBS, patients may have apraxic speech (abnormal prosody, slow speaking rate, repetitions, and prolongations) in association with nonfluent aphasia,[40] but these can sometimes be presenting signs. Regarding oculomotor disturbances, patients with CBS, unlike PSP, do not have ophthalmoplegia until the late stage, but they can have hesitancy in generating a saccade, which can be misinterpreted as ophthalmoplegia. In addition to the aforementioned cortical signs, patients suffering from CBS do not show other peculiar nonmotor symptoms.[40] Neuroimaging can help in the diagnosis of CBD, pointing out asymmetrical cortical fronto-parietal atrophy on MRI, associated with hypometabolism on functional neuroimaging.

DEMENTIA WITH LEWY BODIES

Dementia with Lewy bodies (DLB), like PD and MSA, is an α-synucleinopathy characterized by dementia preceding parkinsonism or developing within 1 year from the onset of parkinsonism.[42] DLB is the second most common form of dementia in elderly people after Alzheimer disease (AD); the core features include fluctuating cognition and recurrent visual hallucinations. Furthermore, patients with DLB exhibit sleep disturbances (RBD), dysautonomia (marked orthostatic hypotension), akinetic-rigid features, and marked sensitivity to D_2-receptor blocking agents, with a rapid induction or worsening of parkinsonism.[43] Neuroimaging can help distinguish DLB from AD (showing reduced striatal uptake on DaTSCAN) and from MSA (showing cardiac denervation at MIBG scintigraphy). Functional studies may show a typical hypometabolism within the occipital cortex.[44]

VASCULAR PARKINSONISM

Vascular parkinsonism (VP), a parkinsonian syndrome that is associated with cerebrovascular disease, is characterized by a sudden onset and continuously progressive stepwise deterioration. Bradykinesia can vary in distribution and severity; the typical phenotype of VP is the so-called "lower-body parkinsonism," in which lower limbs are predominantly affected with impaired balance and gait and disproportionate sparing of the upper limbs. Rigidity is usually of a mixed type (spasticity and rigidity combined) and is often associated with paratonia; resting tremor is usually absent.

Nonmotor disturbances, especially cognitive abnormalities, are not specific for VP. Neuroimaging can play a pivotal role in detecting subcortical vascular lesions associated with VP, even if imaging should be consistent with the peculiar clinical features.[45,46]

SUMMARY

Parkinsonism is one of the most common neurologic disorders in the aging population. Although PD is the most common cause, there is a lengthy differential diagnosis. The diagnosis of PD hinges on recognizing its typical features, including bradykinesia, cogwheel rigidity, rest tremor, unilateral onset, beneficial and sustained response to levodopa. Equally important is to be familiar with the "red flags," which are features not expected with PD and suggest an alternative diagnosis, usually a parkinsonian syndrome. Among others, the important red flags include rapid progression, early falls, early dementia, early hallucinations and delusions, early autonomic failure, early bulbar dysfunction, supranuclear vertical ophthalmoplegia, and especially the lack of a robust response to levodopa, which suggest a parkinsonian syndrome. In general, it is best to have the diagnosis confirmed by a neurologist, especially one with expertise in movement disorders.

DISCLOSURE

The authors have nothing to disclose.

REFERENCES

1. Marsili L, Rizzo G, Colosimo C. Diagnostic criteria for Parkinson's disease: from James Parkinson to the concept of prodromal disease. Front Neurol 2018;9:156.
2. Hughes AJ, Daniel SE, Ben Shlomo Y, et al. The accuracy of diagnosis of Parkinsonian syndromes in a specialist movement disorder service. Brain 2002;125: 861–70.
3. Horstink M, Tolosa E, Bonuccelli U, et al. Review of the therapeutic management of Parkinson's disease. Report of a joint task force of the European Federation of Neurological Societies and the Movement Disorder Society-European Section. Part I: early (uncomplicated) Parkinson's disease. Eur J Neurol 2006;13:1170–85.
4. Horstink M, Tolosa E, Bonuccelli U, et al. Review of the therapeutic management of Parkinson's disease. Report of a joint task force of the European Federation of Neurological Societies and the Movement Disorder Society-European Section. Part II: late (complicated) Parkinson's disease. Eur J Neurol 2006;13:1186–11202.
5. Berardelli A, Wenning GK, Antonini A, et al. EFNS/MDS-ES/ENS [corrected] recommendations for the diagnosis of Parkinson's disease. Eur J Neurol 2013;20: 16–34.
6. Gibb WR, Lees AJ. The relevance of the Lewy body to the pathogenesis of idiopathic Parkinson's disease. J Neurol Neurosurg Psychiatry 1988;51:745–52.
7. Postuma RB, Berg D, Stern M, et al. MDS clinical diagnostic criteria for Parkinson's disease. Mov Disord 2015;30(12):1591–601.
8. Quinn N. Multiple system atrophy–the nature of the beast. J Neurol Neurosurg Psychiatry 1989;(Suppl):78–89.
9. Bhidayasiri R, Sringean J, Reich SG, et al. Red flags phenotyping: a systematic review on clinical features in atypical parkinsonian disorders. Parkinsonism Relat Disord 2019;59:82–92.
10. Colosimo C. The differential diagnosis of parkinsonism: a clinical approach. In: Colosimo C, Riley DE, Wenning GK, editors. Handbook of atypical parkinsonism. Cambridge University Press; 2011. p. 126–41.
11. Fahn S, Kang UJ. Parkinson disease. In: Louis ED, Mayer SA, Lewys P, editors. Merrit's neurology. 13th edition. Cambridge (MA): Wolters Kluwer; 2016. p. 704–21.
12. Haubenberger D, Hallett M. Essential tremor. N Engl J Med 2018;378(19):1802–10.
13. Kim SD, Allen NE, Canning CG, et al. Postural instability in patients with Parkinson's disease. Epidemiology, pathophysiology and management. CNS Drugs 2013;27(2):97–112.

14. Bertram KL, Stirpe P, Colosimo C. Treatment of camptocormia with botulinum toxin. Treatment of camptocormia with botulinum toxin. Toxicon 2015;107(Pt A): 148–53.

15. Okuma Y. Freezing of gait and falls in Parkinson's disease. J Parkinsons Dis 2014; 4(2):255–60.

16. Fahn S, Elton RL, UPDRS Program Members. Unified Parkinson's disease rating scale. In: Fahn S, Marsden CD, Goldstein M, et al, editors. Recent developments in Parkinson's disease, vol. 2. Florham Park (NJ): Macmillan Healthcare Information; 1987. p. 153–63, 293-304.

17. Ramaker C, Marinus J, Stiggelbout AM, et al. Systematic evaluation of rating scales for impairment and disability in Parkinson's disease. Mov Disord 2002; 17:867–76.

18. Goetz CG, Tilley BC, Shaftman SR, et al. Movement disorder society-sponsored revision of the Unified Parkinson's disease rating scale (MDS-UPDRS): scale presentation and clinimetric testing results. Mov Disord 2008;23(15):2129–70.

19. Colosimo C, Martínez-Martín P, Fabbrini G, et al. Task force report on scales to assess dyskinesia in Parkinson's disease: critique and recommendations. Mov Disord 2010;25(9):1131–42.

20. Schapira AHV, Chaudhuri KR, Jenner P. Non-motor features of Parkinson disease. Nat Rev Neurosci 2017;18(8):509.

21. Stirpe P, Hoffman M, Badiali D, et al. Constipation: an emerging risk factor for Parkinson's disease? Eur J Neurol 2016;23(11):1606–13.

22. Colosimo C, Bhidayasiri R. Nonmotor symptoms in Parkinson's disease: are we still waiting for the honeymoon? Eur J Neurol 2016;23(11):1595–6.

23. Barone P, Antonini A, Colosimo C, et al. The PRIAMO study: a multicenter assessment of nonmotor symptoms and their impact on quality of life in Parkinson's disease. Mov Disord 2009;24(11):1641–9.

24. Picillo M, Palladino R, Barone P, et al. The PRIAMO study: urinary dysfunction as a marker of disease progression in early Parkinson's disease. Eur J Neurol 2017; 24(6):788–95.

25. Cossu G, Rinaldi R, Colosimo C. The rise and fall of impulse control behavior disorders. Parkinsonism Relat Disord 2018;46(S1):S24–9.

26. Wennng GK, Fanciulli A. Multiple system atrophy. Springer-Verlag Wien; 2014.

27. Wenning GK, Ben Shlomo Y, Magalhães M, et al. Clinical features and natural history of multiple system atrophy. An analysis of 100 cases. Brain 1994;117(4): 835–45.

28. Colosimo C, Albanese A, Hughes AJ, et al. Some specific clinical features differentiate multiple system atrophy (striatonigral variety) from Parkinson's disease. Arch Neurol 1995;52(3):294–8.

29. Tuite PJ, Krawczewski K. Parkinsonism: a review-of-systems approach to diagnosis. Semin Neurol 2007;27(2):113–22.

30. Quinn NP. How to diagnose multiple system atrophy. Mov Disord 2005;20S2:S5–10.

31. Ghorayeb I, Bioulac B, Tison F. Sleep disorders in multiple system atrophy. J Neural Transm (Vienna) 2005;112(12):1669–75.

32. Steele JC, Richardson JC, Olsewski J. Progressive supranuclear palsy. A heterogeneous degeneration involving the brain stem, basal ganglia and cerebellum with vertical gaze and pseudobulbar palsy, nuchal dystonia and dementia. Arch Neurol 1964;10:333–59.

33. Colosimo C, Fabbrini F, Berardelli A. Progressive supranuclear palsy. In: Colosimo C, Riley DE, Wenning GK, editors. Handbook of atypical parkinsonism. Cambridge, UK: Cambridge University Press; 2011. p. 58–74.

34. Höglinger GU, Respondek G, Stamelou M, et al. Clinical diagnosis of progressive supranuclear palsy: the movement disorder society criteria. Mov Disord 2017; 32(6):853–64.

35. Matsuo H, Takashima H, Kishikawa M, et al. Pure akinesia: an atypical manifestation of progressive supranuclear palsy. J Neurol Neurosurg Psychiatry 1991; 54(5):397–400.

36. Litvan I, Campbell G, Mangone CA, et al. Which clinical features differentiate progressive supranuclear palsy (Steele-Richardson-Olszewski syndrome) from related disorders? A clinicopathological study. Brain 1997;120(Pt 1):65–74.

37. Rivaud-Péchoux S, Vidailhet M, Gallouedec G, et al. Longitudinal ocular motor study in corticobasal degeneration and progressive supranuclear palsy. Neurology 2000;54(5):1029–32.

38. Quattrone A, Nicoletti G, Messina D, et al. MR imaging index for differentiation of progressive supranuclear palsy from Parkinson disease and the Parkinson variant of multiple system atrophy. Radiology 2008;246(1):214–21.

39. Armstrong MJ, Litvan I, Lang AE, et al. Criteria for the diagnosis of corticobasal degeneration. Neurology 2013;80(5):496–503.

40. Armstrong MJ, Lang AE. Corticobasal degeneration. In: Colosimo C, Riley DE, Wenning GK, editors. Handbook of atypical parkinsonism. Cambridge, UK: Cambridge University Press; 2011. p. 75–98.

41. Doody RS, Jankovic J. The alien hand and related signs. J Neurol Neurosurg Psychiatry 1992;55(9):806–10.

42. McKeith IG, Boeve BF, Dickson DW, et al. Diagnosis and management of dementia with Lewy bodies: fourth consensus report of the DLB Consortium. Neurology 2017;89(1):88–100.

43. Barone P, Pellecchia MT, Amboni M. Parkinson's disease and the spectrum of Lewy body disease. In: Colosimo C, Riley DE, Wenning GK, editors. Handbook of atypical parkinsonism. Cambridge, UK: Cambridge University Press; 2011. p. 10–26.

44. Sezgin M, Bilgic B, Tinaz S, et al. Parkinson's disease dementia and Lewy body disease. Semin Neurol 2019;39(2):274–82.

45. Caproni S, Colosimo C. Movement disorders and cerebrovascular diseases: from pathophysiology to treatment. Expert Rev Neurother 2017;17(5):509–19.

46. Vizcarra JA, Lang AE, Sethi KD, et al. Vascular parkinsonism: deconstructing a syndrome. Mov Disord 2015;30(7):886–94.

Does This Patient Have Parkinson Disease or Essential Tremor?

Stephen G. Reich, MD

KEYWORDS

- Tremor • Essential tremor • Parkinson disease

KEY POINTS

- In the elderly patient with tremor, the differential diagnosis is usually between essential tremor (ET) and Parkinson disease (PD).
- It is important to take a careful medication history in the patient with tremor, in particular, exposure to dopamine-blocking medications, which can cause drug-induced parkinsonism.
- ET is a bilateral action tremor of the upper limbs present with maintenance of posture and with movement.
- PD begins unilaterally/asymmetrically, so tremor of 1 hand is likely PD.
- A handwriting sample can distinguish PD from ET. In the former (when the dominant hand is affected), handwriting is small but without tremor. In ET, the handwriting is of normal size but tremulous as is a spiral.

Tremor, defined as a rhythmic oscillation of a body part,[1] is a common symptom in the geriatric population. Although there is a long list of causes of tremor, in older patients, the differential diagnosis almost always boils down to, Is it Parkinson disease (PD) or essential tremor (ET)? Both types of tremor increase in incidence and prevalence with age. PD affects as many as 3% of octogenarians[2] and the prevalence of ET reaches 5% with advancing age.[3] Although tremor is the most common presenting symptom of PD, approximately one-third of people with PD do not have tremor. After reading this article, the reader should be able to distinguish PD from ET. I briefly discuss some other tremors to consider in the elderly, such as drug-induced tremor, dystonic tremor, and orthostatic tremor (OT). Hyperthyroidism should be considered in all patients with tremor but it is uncommon to present with tremor as the main symptom. Wilson disease is rare but an important consideration in the younger patient with tremor but not in the older patient.

Department of Neurology, University of Maryland School of Medicine, 110 South Paca Street, 3rd Floor, Baltimore, MD 21201, USA
E-mail address: sreich@som.umaryland.edu

Clin Geriatr Med 36 (2020) 25–34
https://doi.org/10.1016/j.cger.2019.09.015
0749-0690/20/© 2019 Elsevier Inc. All rights reserved.

The distinction between tremor due to PD versus ET relies almost exclusively on the history and physical examination (**Table 1**).[4–6] One of the most helpful first questions to ask is, How long has the tremor has been present? Most people with PD present within 1 year of onset of tremor whereas patients with ET, because it begins and progresses more insidiously, often have a history of being symptomatic for years or decades, even back to childhood.[7] By definition, according the International Parkinson and Movement Disorder Society (IPMDS), to diagnose ET, it must be present for at least 3 years[1] but that is usually the case when a patient is initially seen. Next, ask, Is there is a family history of tremor? Approximately 15% of people with PD have a positive family history, but this is much more common in ET, reaching approximately 60%, and typically with an autosomal dominant inheritance.[8] Some people with ET say that a family member had PD but because the 2 types of tremor often are confused, clarify the features of the tremor in the relative to see if PD was an appropriate fit. Asking about the response to alcohol can also help distinguish ET from PD because ET often improves transiently after a small amount of alcohol, which usually does not attenuate the tremor of PD. Take a careful drug history because many medications enhance the physiologic tremor, which can mimic ET, and parkinsonism may be drug induced.[9–11] As discussed later, ask which body part(s) is/are affected and if there are any other symptoms, particularly directed to PD, such as slowness, difficulty getting up from a low chair, change in voice, imbalance, difficulty walking, or drooling, none of which should be present in ET.

One of the most important features that distinguishes PD from ET is whether the tremor begins unilaterally or bilaterally. PD typically begins in 1 hand (less commonly in 1 foot), unrelated to handedness, and with time usually spreads to

Table 1
Distinguishing Parkinson disease from essential tremor

Feature	Parkinson Disease	Essential Tremor
Usual duration of symptoms prior to medical contact	6–12 mo	Usually several years or more
Family history	Generally negative (5%–15% with an affected first degree relative)	Often positive (>60%), autosomal dominant
Response to small amount of alcohol	Little or none	Often improves
Position of maximal activation	Rest	Maintenance of posture or with movement
Frequency	3–6 Hz	6–12 Hz
Morphology	Pill-rolling	Flexion-extension
Onset	Unilateral	Bilateral
Body part(s) affected	Upper limb, lower limb, chin, lips, or tongue	Upper limb, head, voice,
Handwriting	Micrographic, atremulous	Normal size, tremulous
Associated signs (bradykinesia, hypomimia, etc.)	Present	Absent

the ipsilateral lower limb and then the opposite side of the body. A helpful clinical point is that early PD is hemi-PD. In contrast, ET, by definition, is a bilateral tremor of the upper limbs and, although some patients may state that the tremor is unilateral, on examination it is bilateral but often asymptomatic in the nondominant limb. The frequency of PD is slower than ET (3–6 Hz vs 6–12 Hz) but this can be difficult to estimate at the bedside, and, because there is overlap, frequency is not a practical way to make the distinction. In contrast, the position of maximal activation does distinguish ET from PD. Essential tremor is defined as a bilateral action tremor of the upper limbs.[1] It is present with maintenance of posture and with movement, the later referred to as a simple kinetic tremor in that the amplitude of ET does not increase as a target is approached, in contrast to intention tremor, reflecting cerebellar disease.[1]

The postural component of ET often is observed best when patients put their hands in front of their nose, not touching, with the elbows elevated in a position, "like you are making wings." Having a patient perform the finger-nose-finger test brings out the kinetic component of ET. The amplitude of ET may not be the same with maintenance of posture and during movement; when the latter is more prominent, it may be mistaken for an intention tremor, because it is not well appreciated that ET is both a postural and kinetic tremor. As discussed previously, the amplitude of intention tremor crescendos as the target is approached and almost always is accompanied by other cerebellar signs (gait ataxia, dysarthria, dysmetria, incoordination, and nystagmus), which are not present in ET, because it is defined by the absence of any abnormalities on examination aside from tremor, that is, an isolated tremor syndrome according to the consensus guideline of the IPMDS.[1]

In contrast to ET, which is a postural and kinetic tremor, PD is a resting tremor, and as discussed previously, it typically is unilateral at onset. It is best observed with the patient relaxing the upper limbs in the lap. If not apparent, it often can be brought out by having the patient perform a distracting task, such as saying the months of the year backwards or doing serial 7s. The classic tremor of PD is referred to as a pill-rolling tremor, looking as though a pill is being rolled between the thumb and other fingers; there also may be flexion and extension at the wrist or pronation-supination of the forearm, both when the limb is a repose. The tremor of PD usually suppresses with movement and with maintenance of posture but after latency of 5 seconds to 10 seconds may reappear during posture, having the same frequency and morphology as the rest tremor, and this is known as a re-emergent tremor and should not be confused with ET despite conflicting with the dictum that PD is a rest tremor.[12] Other less appreciated rule-breakers about PD and ET, which can create diagnostic confusion, are discussed later. A tremor of the hand that persists while a patient is walking is a clue that it is due to PD rather than ET.

As discussed previously, by definition, ET affects both upper limbs but also may affect other parts of the body, most commonly the voice and head, the latter causing either a yes-yes or no-no pattern of shaking.[1] Yet, the diagnosis of ET of the head or voice can be made only in the presence of ET of the upper limbs. Tremor of either the head or voice without tremor of the upper limbs is termed an isolated tremor[1] but is usually the result of dystonia,[13] which can be predominantly tremulous; dystonic tremor is discussed later. Dystonic tremor of the head is termed cervical dystonia (torticollis being the older term) and dystonia affecting the larynx is due to either abnormal adduction of the vocal cords, known as adductor spasmodic dysphonia, or abductor spasm, known as abductor spasmodic dysphonia. But for the purposes of distinguish ET from PD, the point is that tremor of the head or voice points away from PD. In contrast, PD tremor may affect the tongue, chin, jaw, or lower limb and may even start in 1 foot rather than the upper limb, but again, recognize the pattern of unilateral onset, which is the main clue that a tremor is due to PD.

So far, it has been discussed that the position of maximal activation, the onset of the tremor (unilateral or bilateral), and body parts involved are key features to distinguish ET from PD. Another acid test is a handwriting sample and drawing of a spiral. When PD affects the dominant hand, the handwriting becomes small and this symptom and sign alone often is enough to feel confident of the diagnosis. When testing writing, it is important to have patients write (in cursive) a sentence rather than their name. The latter often is overlearned and less effected whereas the micrographia often is apparent only at the end of a sentence or a long word. Although small, the writing in PD is not tremulous because the PD tremor typically suppresses with action. In ET, the handwriting is normal is size but shows evidence of tremor as does a spiral (**Fig. 1**).

In addition to the features of the tremor itself, the ultimate distinction between ET and PD hinges on the presence or absence of other signs. In PD, the hallmark additional sign is bradykinesia, which is not present in ET, nor is rigidity. Bradykinesia is observed in the hand (or foot) affected by tremor when a patient is asked to make rapid, repetitive movements, such as touching the tips of the index finger and thumb, opening and closing the hand, and tapping the toe or heel, demonstrating a decremental response, that is diminishing amplitude with continuous movement and/or hesitation of movement.[14] Rigidity is felt by passively moving a limb, producing a ratchety or cogwheel-type resistance. Other features of early PD include diminished blink rate, facial expression, voice volume, and intonation. There often is mild difficulty arising from a chair, diminished arm swing, initially on 1 side (often, as discussed previously, with tremor), a slow gait with mild shuffling, mildly flexed posture, and possibly impaired balance on the pull test, but this sign typically is seen in more advanced PD rather than at presentation.

For diagnosis of ET, there should be no additional signs; hence, the traditional designation of ET as a monosymptomatic disorder. Yet, within the past 2 decades, it has become appreciated that ET may not be as isolated as has been thought, and this evolving concept has been led mainly by the work of Dr Elan Louis.[4,15] In addition to tremor, some patients demonstrate other neurologic soft signs, such as subtle

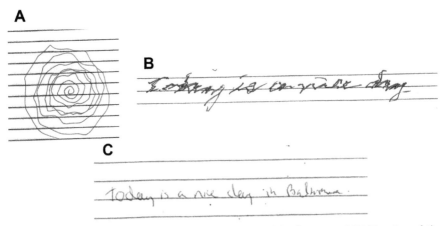

Fig. 1. The spiral (*A*) and top sentence (*B*) demonstrate the features of ET. The size of the handwriting is normal but tremulous. The bottom sample of handwriting (*C*), from a patient with PD, starts off normal-sized but becomes micrographic at the end of the sentence. ([*B*] *From* Reich SG. Essential tremor. Med Clin North Am. 2019;103(2):352; with permission.)

dystonia, not thought to be sufficient for a diagnosis of dystonic tremor, imbalance with gait ataxia, and cognitive impairment. To recognize cases of ET that are not isolated, the IPMDS carved out a separate category known as ET plus.[1,16] The debate and controversy about the role of other signs in patients with ET notwithstanding, for the purposes of geriatricians seeing a patient with suspected ET, any neurologic signs other than tremor should trigger a consultation with a neurologist and preferably a specialist in movement disorders.

JUST WHEN YOU THOUGHT YOU COULD DISTINGUISH PARKINSON DISEASE FROM ESSENTIAL TREMOR
Some Exceptions to the Rules

Following the guidelines discussed previously, summarized in **Table 1**, there should be little difficulty distinguishing PD from ET. Yes, as discussed, there are a few exceptions to the rules that are potential diagnostic pitfalls. Although PD is a rest tremor, the same tremor may appear after maintaining posture for 5 seconds to 10 seconds. Because this tremor has the same frequency and morphology as the tremor at rest, it is referred to as a re-emergent tremor[12] and should not dissuade from diagnosing PD. Many people with PD, if examined carefully, have a slightly faster, bilateral postural tremor, which is usually not symptomatic; it is subtle and not likely to be confused with ET.[17]

Although PD and ET are separate disorders, there is overlap.[18] It is not too uncommon to see a patient for the recent onset of a unilateral rest tremor, with other signs of typical PD, but who gives a history of tremor of both limbs going back decades, indicating preexisting ET with superimposed PD and both types of tremor present on examination. There are 4 reasons why patients with ET may demonstrate a rest tremor. First, they may not be completely at rest and even a slight degree of muscle activation elicits tremor that disappears as the limb relaxes completely. Second, it is well appreciated that patients with long-standing ET may develop an actual rest tremor with the features of a parkinsonian tremor but without other signs of PD. Third, some patients with ET may have a mild tremor of the proximal lower extremities and the hand appears to shake simply because it is resting on a tremulous thigh; that there is no actual resting tremor can be proved by having patients rest a hand on the armrest of the chair. Lastly, some patients with ET eventually develop clear PD and it remains an area of controversy about whether ET is a risk factor for PD.[18]

What Is a DaTscan™ and When Should It Be Ordered?

A DaTscan is an imaging technique using single-photon emission computer tomography to determine the concentration of the radiopharmaceutical (^{123}ioflupane) binding to the presynaptic dopamine transporter in the striatum. In the presence of nigrostriatal dopaminergic degeneration, the concentration of the presynaptic dopamine transporter declines, leading to diminished uptake.[19] This originally was approved to distinguish PD, in which there is diminished binding, from ET with normal binding. Yet, with rare exceptions, the distinction between PD and ET can be made on clinical grounds and additional testing is not necessary. In answer to the question, When should I order a DaTscan? my answer to a geriatrician, admitting my bias, is, never.[20] If it is unclear whether a patient has PD or ET, the appropriate next step is referral to a neurologist and ideally one specializing in movement disorders.

Although a DaTscan is not needed to distinguish ET from PD, there are other off-label indications when a DaTscan can be useful, mainly for distinguishing whether a patient's parkinsonism is associated with nigrostriatal degeneration. Examples of where it is not include drug-induced parkinsonism and parkinsonism mimicked by normal pressure hydrocephalus, multiple strokes, normal aging, and a functional disorder. A DaTscan is unable to distinguish PD from other causes of parkinsonism associated with nigrostriatal degeneration, such as multiple system atrophy or progressive supranuclear palsy.[21]

How Can Parkinson Disease and Essential Tremor Be Treated?

The treatment of PD is covered in Management of Early Parkinson Disease & Management of Motor Features in Advanced Parkinson Disease. With regard to a parkinsonian tremor, for many people this is not a particularly problematic symptom because it usually attenuates with use of the limb. Some patients find it embarrassing and that alone may justify treatment. Antiparkinsonian medications tend to be less effective for tremor, in particular, large amplitude tremor, than for the other cardinal signs of PD. Patients should be counseled that medical therapy will not make the tremor resolve but, instead, they should anticipate improvement. In older patients with PD, I rely predominantly on levodopa because it is the most effective and best tolerated of the antiparkinsonian medications. There is a long-standing belief that anticholinergics are more effective for tremor but that has not been established and this class of medications is best to avoid in the elderly due to side effects, including dry mouth, constipation, urinary retention, blurred vision, impaired concentration, memory, and confusion. For patients with disabling PD tremor that does not improve sufficiently with medication, either deep brain stimulation (DBS) or focused ultrasound (discussed later) can be considered.

For patients with ET, the first step is to determine if treatment is needed. Many patients with ET present fearing they have PD and for them, when there is not physical limitation from the tremor, reassurance and education may be all that is needed. The decision about treatment requires a careful discussion with patients about how they are impacted by ET. Common problems include difficulty writing, using eating utensils, using tools such as a screwdriver, drinking from a cup, pouring liquid, holding a book or newspaper, applying makeup, and fastening jewelry. Some patients are embarrassed by tremor (especially ET tremor of the head or voice) and often are too embarrassed to admit this so need to be asked directly. ET of the head often is asymptomatic and rarely causes any physical limitation. ET of the voice may interfere with communication.

If treatment is needed, and this refers to upper limb tremor, then there are evidence-based guidelines available to direct treatment. The first was published by the American Academy of Neurology in 2005[22] and gave A-level recommendations to primidone, propranolol, and propranolol LA. B-level recommendations were given to alprazolam, atenolol, gabapentin, sotalol, and topiramate. The following were given C-level recommendations: clonazepam, clozapine, nadolol, nimodipine, and botulinum toxin for tremor of the upper limb, head, and voice and DBS of the thalamus and thalamotomy. An update based on interval studies was published in 2011[23] and there were no new agents qualifying for A-level recommendations; instead, several prior recommendations were downgraded, including the recommendation that levetiracetam and 3,4-diaminopyridine should not be used, and, similarly flunarizine, with insufficient evidence to recommend pregabalin, zonisamide, or clozapine.

More recently, the IPDMDS published an evidence-based review with the top level being efficacious followed by likely efficacious.[24] Similar to the American Academy of Neurology guideline, propranolol and primidone were found to be efficacious along with topiramate at a daily dose greater than 200 mg. Likely efficacious recommendations, again referring to upper limb tremor, were given for alprazolam, botulinum toxin type A, unilateral DBS of the thalamus, unilateral thalamotomy, and unilateral focused ultrasound.

From a practical standpoint, when a patient with ET needs to be treated, the first choice is between propranolol and primidone and they are equally efficacious. To assess the effect of treatment, it is useful to have a patient follow the effect on 2 or 3 activities that they consider most affected. If there are no contraindications, propranolol should be started in older patients at a low dose, such as 10 mg or 20 mg twice per day, and escalated slowly until the tremor improves to a degree that allows patients to function at a more acceptable level and there are no problematic side effects. It is important to counsel patients that the tremor will not go away. Typical effective doses are from 60 mg to 180 mg per day; younger patients may have a higher tolerance. Once a stable dose of propranolol is reached, patients can be converted to the long acting preparation for ease of administration.

If primidone is chosen as the first-line treatment, then it should be started at 25 mg at night. Some patients experience the first-dose phenomenon, feeling dizzy, nauseated, sleepy, and off balance the day after taking the first dose but warning them that this may happen and that it is transient and self-limited generally allows for continuing therapy. Many people can take primidone once per day but I often split the dose, aiming for an initial dose of 50 mg twice per day, achieved by a slow escalation over several weeks. From there, based on the results and presence of side effects (many of which improve with time), the dose can be escalated slowly. Although the maximal dose is 750 mg per day, most of the benefit is achieved at 300 mg to 400 mg per day and there often is little to be gained after that. If the maximally tolerated dose of either propranolol or primidone is not sufficiently beneficial, they should be combined because the effect is synergistic. Elderly patients may not be able to tolerate a therapeutic dose of either but improve with a low dose of propranolol and primidone.

If propranolol and primidone are not effective, then the likelihood that a second-tier medication, especially in the elderly, will be effective and well tolerated is low. Gabapentin or topiramate are considerations but most older patients cannot tolerate the dose of topiramate (>200 mg) needed. At this point, many elderly patients acquiesce to living with the tremor. An evaluation by an occupational therapist is worth pursuing because some patients benefit from suggestions, such as weighted utensils, among others.

In those whose tremor is sufficiently debilitating, that it is not feasible to put up with it, the next options include either unilateral thalamotomy, unilateral or bilateral DBS, or the newer therapy of focused ultrasound,[24] which can only be performed unilaterally. At this point, patients should be referred to a center with expertise in these options. Just like medical therapy, the surgical options (recognizing that focused ultrasound is invasive but not really surgical), each has its benefits and drawbacks. With the advent of DBS[25] (best thought of as putting a pacemaker in the brain rather than the heart), radiofrequency thalamotomy has largely been abandoned. DBS of the ventral intermediate nucleus of thalamus has the advantage of being able to be performed bilaterally because for many patients with ET, unilateral improvement is insufficient. An additional advantage is that the stimulation parameters can be adjusted to optimize benefit and keep pace with additional progression of tremor with time. It requires chronic hardware and follow-up visits to program the impulse pulse generator. DBS has been used for more than 25 years, so has a well-established track record of prolonged benefit. Potential complications include a very low risk of intracerebral hemorrhage and infection of the hardware.

Magnetic resonance imaging–guided focused ultrasound,[26–28] at the present time, can be performed only unilaterally and, therefore, is a good option for patients who would be satisfied to have improvement in only the dominant hand tremor. The benefit is immediate and no hardware or adjustments are required but, as a more recent treatment, it does not have the long-term efficacy data of DBS. Like DBS, there is a low rate of complications, especially serious complications (1.6%), and most are mild and transient, including numbness or imbalance.[29]

SOME OTHER TYPES OF TREMOR IN THE ELDERLY
Drug-induced Tremor

Although tremor in the elderly patient is usually due to ET or PD, there are a few other types of tremor that geriatricians should be familiar with. The first is drug-induced tremor.[9–11] This causes 2 types of tremor. The first is an enhanced physiologic tremor manifested by a postural and kinetic tremor of the upper limbs, which may resemble ET but typically is a bit faster (8–12 Hz) and of low amplitude.[1] Most patients with a drug-induced enhanced physiologic tremor are asymptomatic or only minimally symptomatic. Many commonly used drugs in the elderly can cause tremor, including lithium, valproic acid, sympathomimetics, corticosteroids, antidepressants, amiodarone, neuroleptics, immunosuppressants, and chemotherapeutic agents, among others. Only if the tremor is problematic should discontinuation of the offended drug be considered and, if that is not feasible, then a β-blocker can be considered.

The second type of drug-induced tremor is parkinsonism.[11] Although drug-induced parkinsonism is usually atremulous, it can manifest with a typical parkinsonian resting tremor, which may be unilateral and look just like PD. It is due to antidopaminergic medications, including antipsychotics and antiemetics (metoclopramide). Although it is well appreciated that first-generation antipsychotics can cause drug-induced parkinsonism and tardive syndromes, it is less well appreciated that almost all of the second-generation antispychotics can do the same. It is important to take a careful drug history in any patient with parkinsonism. Drug-induced parkinsonism may take up to 1 year to resolve after the offending medication is stopped and, therefore, patients may no longer be on the medication at the time of presentation.

Dystonic Tremor

Dystonia is a movement disorder characterized by sustained or intermittent, stereotyped muscle contractions. Dystonia typically causes abnormal postures and twisting movements but often is tremulous.[30,31] Sometimes the tremor of dystonia is so prominent that it grabs all the attention and a subtle degree of dystonia is not appreciated. The 2 types of dystonic tremor that geriatricians should be familiar with are cervical dystonia and laryngeal dystonia. The former is characterized by an abnormal position of the head, including turning, tilting, pulling backward or forward, or a combination. Many patients with cervical dystonia have only the spasm but there often is a coexistent tremor of the head. A dystonic tremor, unlike ET of the head, tends to be more jerky and usually is not a regular oscillation and exacerbates when patients attempt to move their head opposite of the direction due to dystonia. So, if a tremor of the head is seen, look carefully for dystonia. Recall that ET of the head can be diagnosed only when there is ET of the upper limbs.

The other type of dystonic tremor to be familiar with is laryngeal dystonia. The takes 2 forms. The first, adductor spasmodic dysphonia, is due to adductor spasm of the vocal cords producing a strained voice with irregular breaks as though the person is being strangled. In contrast, abductor spasmodic dysphonia causes a breathy voice as though the person is attempting to speak after running up a flight of stairs.

Orthostatic Tremor

OT is a rare tremor that generally occurs in the middle-aged to older patient. It manifests as a low-amplitude, very rapid (13–18 Hz) tremor of both lower extremities only while standing.[1,32] It often presents a diagnostic challenge because patients usually do not complain or even recognize tremor but instead report that standing is difficult, uncomfortable, or associated with a sense of weakness of the lower extremities or they feel imbalance. For some patients, the tremor is so unpleasant that they become phobic of standing and may be incorrectly diagnosed as having a functional disorder. The diagnosis should be suspected from the unique history of difficulty standing but no difficulty walking. On examination, while standing, there is a subtle, rapid tremor of the lower extremities. Sometimes this can be seen but, if not, it can be palpated or even heard through the stethoscope. It has a characteristic sound of the rotor of a helicopter, hence the helicopter sign.[33] The remainder of the examination is normal but there may be associated tremor in other parts of the body. The definite test for OT is an electromyogram to confirm the presence of a rapid tremor.

Because OT is an uncommon disorder and incompletely understood, treatment is largely empirical because there are no controlled trials. Options include clonazepam, propranolol, primidone, gabapentin, and levetiracetam.

DISCLOSURE STATEMENT

The author has nothing to disclose.

REFERENCES

1. Bhatia KP, Bain P, Bajaj N, et al. Consensus statement on the classification of tremors. From the task force on tremor of the International Parkinson and movement disorder Society. Mov Disord 2018;33:75–87.
2. Lee A, Gilbert RM. Epidemiology of Parkinson disease. Neurol Clin 2016;34: 955–65.
3. Louis ED, Ferreira JJ. How common is the most common adult movement disorder? Update on the worldwide prevalence of essential tremor. Mov Disord 2010; 25:534–41.
4. Clark LN, Louis ED. Essential tremor. Handb Clin Neurol 2018;147:229–39.
5. Haubenberger D, Hallett M. Essential tremor. N Engl J Med 2018;19:1802–10.
6. Louis ED. Twelve clinical pearls to help distinguish essential tremor from other tremors. Expert Rev Neurother 2014;14:1057–65.
7. Jankovic J, Madisetty J, Vuong KD. Essential tremor among children. Pediatrics 2004;114:1203–5.
8. Deng H, Le W, Jankovic J. Genetics of essential tremor. Brain 2007;130:1456–64.
9. Morgan JC, Sethi KD. Drug-induced tremors. Lancet Neurol 2005;4:866--76.
10. Factor SA, Burkhard PR, Caroff S, et al. Recent developments in drug-induced movement disorders: a mixed picture. Lancet Neurol 2019;18:880–90.
11. Esper CD, Factor SA. Failure of recognition of drug-induced parkinsonism in the elderly. Mov Disord 2008;23:401–4.
12. Jankovic J, Schwartz KS, Ondo W. Re-emergent tremor of Parkinson's disease. J Neurol Neurosurg Psychiatry 1999;67:646–50.
13. Quinn NP, Schneider SA, Schwingenschuh P, et al. Tremor–some controversial aspects. Mov Disord 2011;26:18–23.

14. Postuma RB, Berg D, Stern M, et al. MDS clinical diagnostic criteria for Parkinson's disease. Mov Disord 2015;30:1591–601.
15. Louis ED. The evolving definition of essential tremor: what are we dealing with? Parkinsonism Relat Disord 2017;46(Suppl 1):S87–91.
16. Louis ED. Essential tremor: "Plus" or "Minus". Perhaps now is the time to adopt the term "the essential tremors". Parkinsonism Relat Disord 2018;56:111–2.
17. Dirkx MF, Zach H, Bloem BR, et al. The nature of postural tremor in Parkinson disease. Neurology 2018;90:e1095–103.
18. Tarakad A, Jankovic J. Essential tremor and Parkinson's disease: exploring the relationship. Tremor Other Hyperkinet Mov 2019;9:1–10.
19. Bajaj N, Hauser RA, Grachev ID. Clinical utility of dopamine transporter single photon emission CT (DaT-SPECT) with (123I) ioflupane in diagnosis of parkinsonian syndromes. J Neurol Neurosurg Psychiatry 2013;84:1288–95.
20. Zimmerman S. All my husband needed was a good physical examination. JAMA Intern Med 2015;175:340.
21. Isaacson SH, Fisher S, Gupta F, et al. Clinical utility of DaTscan™ imaging in the evaluation of patients with parkinsonism: a US perspective. Expert Rev Neurother 2017;17:219–25.
22. Zesiewicz TA, Elble RJ, Louis ED, et al. Practice parameter: therapies for essential tremor. Neurology 2005;64:2008–20.
23. Zesiewicz TA, Elble RJ, Louis ED, et al. Evidence-based guideline update: treatment of essential tremor: report of the Quality Standards subcommittee of the American Academy of Neurology. Neurology 2011;77:1752–5.
24. Ferreira JJ, Mestre TA, Lyons KE, et al. MDS task force on tremor and the MDS evidence based medicine Committee.MDS evidence-based review of treatments for essential tremor. Mov Disord 2019;34:950–8.
25. Nazzaro JM, Lyons KE, Pahwa R. Deep brain stimulation for essential tremor. Handb Clin Neurol 2013;116:155–66.
26. Fishman PS, Frenkel V. Treatment of movement disorders with focused ultrasound. J Cent Nerv Syst Dis 2017;9. 1179573517705670.
27. Fishman PS, Elias WJ, Ghanouni P, et al. A prospective trial of magnetic resonance-guided focused ultrasound thalamotomy for essential tremor: results at the 2-year follow-up. Ann Neurol 2018;83:107–14.
28. Elias WJ, Lipsman N, Ondo WG, et al. A randomized trial of focused ultrasound thalamotomy for essential tremor. N Engl J Med 2016;375:730–9.
29. Fishman PS, Elias WJ, Ghanouni P, et al. Neurological adverse event profile of magnetic resonance imaging-guided focused ultrasound thalamotomy for essential tremor. Mov Disord 2018;33:843–7.
30. Albanese A, Bhatia K, Bressman SB, et al. Phenomenology and classification of dystonia: a consensus update. Mov Disord 2013;28:863–73.
31. Pandey S, Sarma N. Tremor in dystonia. Parkinsonism Relat Disord 2016;29:3–9.
32. Hassan A, Ahlskog JE, Matsumoto JY, et al. Orthostatic tremor: clinical, electrophysiologic, and treatment findings in 184 patients. Neurology 2016;86:458–64.
33. DeOrchis VS, Geyer HL, Herskovitz S. Teaching video neuroimages: orthostatic tremor: the helicopter sign. Neurology 2013;80:e161.

Management of Early Parkinson Disease

Theresa A. Zesiewicz, MD[a,b,c],*, Yarema Bezchlibnyk, MD, PhD[c,d],
Nicolas Dohse, BS[a,b,e,1], Shaila D. Ghanekar[a,b,c,2]

KEYWORDS

- Parkinson disease • Early management • Pharmacology • Exercise
- Deep brain stimulation

KEY POINTS

- Early Parkinson disease may be treated with dopamine agonists, monoamine oxidase B inhibitors, amantadine, or anticholinergic medications. However, patients eventually need to take levodopa to control their symptoms.
- The decision as to when to initiate treatment in early Parkinson disease depends on many factors, including age, employment status, and comorbid conditions.
- Bothersome symptoms that negatively affect quality of life should be treated.

Continued

Disclosure: Dr T.A. Zesiewicz has received personal compensation for serving on the advisory boards of Boston Scientific, Reata Pharmaceuticals, Inc, and Steminent Biotherapeutics; Dr T. A. Zesiewicz has received personal compensation as senior editor for Neurodegenerative Disease Management and as a consultant for Steminent Biotherapeutics; Dr T.A. Zesiewicz has received royalty payments as coinventor of varenicline for treating imbalance (patent number 9,463,190) and nonataxic imbalance (patent number 9,782,404); Dr T.A. Zesiewicz has received research/grant support as principal investigator/investigator for studies from AbbVie, Biogen, Biohaven Pharmaceutics, Boston Scientific, Bukwang Pharmaceuticals Co, Ltd, Cala Health, Inc, Cavion, Friedreich's Ataxia Research Alliance, Houston Methodist Research Institute, National Institutes of Health (READISCA U01), Retrotope Inc, and Takeda Development Center Americas, Inc. The other authors have nothing to disclose.

[a] Department of Neurology, University of South Florida, Ataxia Research Center, Tampa, FL, USA; [b] Frances J. Zesiewicz Foundation for Parkinson Disease; [c] University of South Florida, Movement Disorders Neuromodulation Center, Tampa, FL, USA; [d] Department of Neurosurgery and Brain Repair, University of South Florida, 2 Tampa General Circle STC-7049, Tampa, FL 33606, USA; [e] Sidney Kimmel Medical College, Thomas Jefferson University, Philadelphia, PA, USA
[1] Present address: 726 Market Street, Suite 705, Philadelphia, PA 19106.
[2] Present address: 2625 Hawks Landing Boulevard, Palm Harbor, FL 34685.
* Corresponding author. University of South Florida, 12901 Bruce B. Downs Boulevard, MDC Box 55, Tampa, FL 33612.
E-mail address: tzesiewi@health.usf.edu

Clin Geriatr Med 36 (2020) 35–41
https://doi.org/10.1016/j.cger.2019.09.001
0749-0690/20/Published by Elsevier Inc.

Continued

- The EARLYSTIM (Controlled Trial of Deep Brain Stimulation in Early Patients with Parkinson Disease) study showed improved quality of life in patients earlier in the course of the disease. However, appropriate patient selection, clear diagnosis of levodopa-responsive Parkinson disease, and monitoring of psychological symptoms are important factors to consider with deep brain stimulation surgery.
- Exercise is beneficial for patients with Parkinson disease and should be strongly encouraged but performed safely.

INTRODUCTION

Parkinson disease is a progressive, neurodegenerative disorder that affects millions of people worldwide. The disease is marked by motor and nonmotor symptoms, many of which were described by James Parkinson more than 200 years ago. Parkinson disease results in considerable morbidity and financial strain. The cost of Parkinson disease in terms of lost wages for patients and caregivers alone is estimated to reach billions of dollars.

Parkinson disease remains one of the few neurodegenerative diseases whose symptoms are effectively treated with dopaminergic therapy. However, the so-called early honeymoon phase characterized by clinical benefit eventually transitions to less optimal motor response. The choice of treatment in early Parkinson disease is important, because clinical efficacy of a medication should be weighed against financial considerations, ease of administration, and potential long-term adverse events.

This article reviews pharmacologic and nonpharmacologic treatment of early-stage Parkinson disease.

EARLY PARKINSON DISEASE

The cardinal motor symptoms of Parkinson disease include tremor, bradykinesia, rigidity, and postural instability (impairment of balance). The disease is also marked by nonmotor symptoms, including psychiatric symptoms, sleep disorders, cognitive dysfunction, dysautonomia, and sensory impairment.[1]

The timing as to when levodopa is to be started varies from patient to patient but virtually all patients end up requiring levodopa in order to optimize control of their symptoms. After an initial period of good response to levodopa characterized by a stable therapeutic benefit throughout the day (honeymoon period), patients start experiencing a waning of the effect with each dose of levodopa (wearing off), which requires an increase in the number of daily doses. Early Parkinson disease might be defined as the time period that lasts from the initial appearance of symptoms to the development of these motor fluctuations, which may also include the appearance of involuntary movements known as levodopa-induced dyskinesias.[2]

The underpinnings of Parkinson disease seem to begin much earlier than the first visible symptoms. The Movement Disorder Task Force recognizes 3 stages in early Parkinson disease.[3] The first stage is called the preclinical phase, which marks the onset of neurodegeneration without clinical symptoms; the second stage is the prodromal phase, in which disease symptoms become noticeable but are not yet sufficient to make a diagnosis; the third and final phase is the clinical phase, in which symptoms of Parkinson disease are obvious and recognizable.[3] Although there are currently no neuroprotective or neurorestorative treatments, biomarkers to identify the early preclinical and prodromal phases of the disease will be important to implement neuroprotective strategies.

PHARMACOLOGIC AGENTS FOR EARLY PARKINSON DISEASE

Medications to treat early Parkinson disease include carbidopa/levodopa (immediate and controlled-release forms as well as orally disintegrating tablets and a combination controlled-release/immediate-release formulation), dopamine agonists (pramipexole, ropinirole, rotigotine), monoamine oxidase (MAO) B inhibitors (rasagiline), anticholinergic medications (trihexyphenidyl and benztropine), and a presynaptic dopaminergic medication (amantadine). These medications, as well as some additional ones, are used in more advance disease[4] (see Henry Moore and colleagues' article, "Management of Motor Features in Advanced Parkinson Disease," in this issue).

Levodopa is the gold standard for treating Parkinson disease. Research on levodopa took place in the 1950s and 1960s, when Arvid Carlsson[5] found that levodopa reversed reserpine-induced akinesia, and George Cotzias[6] tested it in a cohort of patients and noted favorable results. Levodopa was eventually paired with carbidopa, a dopa decarboxylase inhibitor, in order to reduce nausea and peripheral breakdown of levodopa. It remains the anchor of Parkinson disease pharmacologic treatment to date, both in early and advanced disease. Levodopa effectively treats bradykinesia and rigidity, but has less robust efficacy for tremor.[7] Side effects of carbidopa/levodopa may include nausea, vomiting, orthostatic hypotension, and neuropsychiatric issues, including hallucinations.[8]

Dopamine agonists are effective as monotherapy and adjunct therapy for Parkinson disease. They directly stimulate postsynaptic dopamine receptors, thereby bypassing degenerating dopamine neurons; they are also known to have longer half-lives than levodopa.[9,10] The immediate formulations are given 3 times daily, whereas pramipexole and ropinirole have extended-release, once-daily formulations. Rotigotine is administered as a transdermal patch.[8,11] Patients who use dopamine agonists as monotherapy eventually require adjunct therapy with levodopa approximately 3 to 5 years after starting treatment.[11]

MAO-B inhibitors are selective and irreversible agents that limit the reuptake of dopamine in the brain and prevent its breakdown. They have moderate efficacy against motor symptoms and may be used as monotherapeutic and adjunct therapeutic agents for Parkinson disease.[12] A rare side effect is the serotonin syndrome, which may occur when these agents are used with certain selective serotonin reuptake inhibitors (SSRIs); however, this syndrome has a significantly lower incidence when SSRIs are coadministered with MAO-B inhibitors rather than MAO or MAO-A inhibitors.[12] In addition to investigations into dopamine agonists for early treatment, clinical trials have been conducted to test the potential benefits of MAO-B inhibitors as neuroprotective agents but results have been inconclusive.[12]

Amantadine, an N-methyl-D-aspartate receptor antagonist, can be used to treat parkinsonian symptoms (it has also been proved useful in advanced Parkinson disease as the only proven antidyskinesia drug). Side effects are generally neuropsychiatric (confusion, hallucinations) or sleep related but also include dizziness, constipation, and livedo reticularis.[9,13]

Anticholinergic medications, including trihexyphenidyl and benztropine, are primarily used to treat tremor in younger patients. Because of their side effects, which include dry mouth, urinary retention, confusion, and constipation, they are generally avoided in elderly patients, particularly those more than 70 years of age.[13]

TREATMENT STRATEGIES IN EARLY PARKINSON DISEASE

Medical management of early Parkinson disease may include treatment of bothersome symptoms, or a watch-and-wait strategy for milder symptoms.[14] Medications provide symptomatic relief, because there are no neuroprotective or neurorestorative therapies currently available. It is generally agreed that patients should be treated if their symptoms impair their quality of life and/or productivity. The choice of initial medication depends on the severity of a patient's symptoms, age, employment status, phenomenology, and comorbid conditions such as cognitive ability or excessive daytime sleepiness. There is no known benefit of withholding treatment from patients who require symptomatic therapy.

Several treatment strategies may be used in early Parkinson disease, including dopamine agonists, MAO-B inhibitors, or anticholinergic medications, and optimizing them as needed. When these medications fail to confer adequate motor benefit, levodopa may be added in what is termed levodopa rescue.[15] In contrast, patients who need tight symptom control in order to continue their employment or activities of daily living, or who develop side effects from nonlevodopa agents, may require levodopa treatment early in the disease.

Younger patients (<60 years of age) with early Parkinson disease often have special considerations to contend with in terms of short-term and long-term treatment strategies. Many patients are still employed or have childcare and eldercare duties that warrant symptomatic benefit. Inadequately treated symptoms may lead to early retirement or lost wages. Initial treatment of younger patients with Parkinson disease may include dopamine agonists, MAO-B inhibitors, levodopa, anticholinergic medications, or no medication, with an emphasis on exercise. Younger patients are also less likely than their elderly counterparts to experience cognitive side effects from dopamine agonists or anticholinergic agents. A prudent approach may include treatment with the lowest dose of levodopa that adequately treats motor symptoms, perhaps starting with 50 mg a day and aiming for 100 mg 3 times a day. In older patients with evidence of cognitive decline, excessive daytime sleepiness, or other comorbid conditions, it may be more appropriate to start initial treatment with levodopa.

LEVODOPA: EARLY VERSUS DELAYED USE

Levodopa is the gold standard for Parkinson disease, but there have been conflicting opinions regarding its use in the early stages of the disease. The decision to use levodopa as early treatment of Parkinson disease in younger patients has been controversial. The association between levodopa and motor fluctuations was made toward the end of the twenty-first century and heralded the arrival of nonlevodopa medications that were designed to delay their onset. Several studies suggested that early treatment of Parkinson disease with a dopamine agonist yielded a lower incidence of motor fluctuations compared with initial treatment with levodopa.[16,17] Higher doses of levodopa have also been associated with an earlier onset of motor fluctuations. The Earlier versus Later Levodopa (ELLDOPA) clinical trial was designed to determine whether levodopa could be safely initiated early in the disease process. De novo patients who received carbidopa-levodopa had significantly lower, or better, clinical scores after 40 weeks of treatment compared with patients who received placebo ($P<.001$).[18] However, patients treated with the highest dosage of levodopa, 50/200 mg 3 times a day, experienced the highest incidence of dyskinesia and other motor complications.[18]

Recent evidence indicates that higher doses of levodopa and longer disease duration probably play more important roles in the onset of motor fluctuations than the duration of levodopa treatment.[19] However, the negative perception of levodopa may cause patients to refuse to use it, because of anxiety about how it may affect them in the future. Patients may choose to accept disabling symptoms just to save levodopa for later. Note that there is no definitive evidence that levodopa induces cell death or leads to further dopaminergic neuronal degeneration.[20] It is essential that practitioners give patients accurate information about the pros and cons of early disease treatment and that the pair arrive at an informative choice together.

NONMOTOR SYMPTOMS

The presence of potential nonmotor symptoms should be discussed at office visits for Parkinson disease at all disease stages. Most patients experience more than 1 nonmotor symptom as part of their disease process, and these are often more disabling than motor symptoms. Nonmotor symptoms have a negative impact on quality of life, even in patients who are newly diagnosed.[21] Negative feelings of well-being may be particularly affected by sleep, neuropsychiatric, and cognitive dysfunction.[21]

SURGICAL TREATMENT OF PARKINSON DISEASE

Deep brain stimulation (DBS) was initially approved by the US Food and Drug Administration (FDA) in 2002 to treat symptoms of advanced Parkinson disease, based on several large multicenter randomized controlled trials showing that DBS within the subthalamic nucleus (STN) or globus pallidus internus significantly improved quality of life, motor fluctuations, bradykinesia, and rigidity, which persisted for up to 10 years.[22] On this basis, most patients present for this therapy 11 to 13 years after the onset of symptoms, with significant disability and prominent motor fluctuations.[22] Such clear efficacy of this intervention in patients with advanced symptoms[23,24] has led to efforts to assess its utility in patients presenting earlier in the course of their disease in an effort to improve quality of life, before deterioration in psychological symptoms and the onset of dopamine-resistant features. These efforts culminated in the EARLYSTIM trial (Controlled Trial of Deep Brain Stimulation in Early Patients with Parkinson Disease), which evaluated quality of life using the Parkinson Disease Questionnaire (PDQ-39).[25] More than 250 patients were randomized to receive STN-DBS and best medical management or best medical treatment alone over a 2-year period. Based on the results of this trial, in 2015, the FDA announced approval for the use of DBS for treatment of Parkinson disease symptoms of at least 4 years' duration, including recent or long-standing complications that are not optimally controlled with medication.

Serious adverse events occurred in almost 55% of patients who received STN compared with 44% of those who received only medical management.[25] However, serious adverse events related to surgical implantation or the neurostimulation device occurred in 17.7% of patients.[25] This finding was comparable with surgical complication rates reported in prior studies on patients with advanced disease.[23,24] In addition, there was a high rate of suicidal behavior, including suicide, which did not differ between treatment groups. However, this finding underscores the need for close monitoring of psychiatric status in patients with Parkinson disease, whether undergoing DBS or not.[24]

The success of DBS depends in part on patient selection and close follow-up in the immediate postoperative period to optimize stimulation parameters and identify deleterious effects of stimulation. These factors are arguably more important in patients with early motor complications from Parkinson disease. Parkinson disease remains a clinical diagnosis and it must be distinguished from other atypical parkinsonisms, which typically manifests in delayed fashion, which may lead to misdiagnosis in patients with early Parkinson disease. Such considerations highlight the importance of clinical experience and well-integrated multidisciplinary teams in the surgical management of patients with early motor fluctuation in Parkinson disease. Thus, caution should be used in generalizing the EARLYSTIM results more broadly, outside of an academic setting.

EXERCISE IN PARKINSON DISEASE

Exercise is an important component for treatment of Parkinson disease at any stage. Patients with Parkinson disease eventually develop dopamine-resistant symptoms, including postural instability and freezing. Core strength training exercises, aerobic training, tai chi, treadmill, balance, yoga, boxing, progressive resistance, and dance and music therapy are types of exercise that may be beneficial. Specific types of exercise regimens may be used to improved various impairments in Parkinson disease.[26] One study found that long-term aerobic exercise may slow the progression of Parkinson disease[27]; another reported that 24 months of structured, supervised exercise provided benefit in functional performance outcomes in patients with moderate Parkinson disease.[26] Progressive resistance exercise has also been found to be a useful adjunct therapy to improve motor symptoms.[28]

SUMMARY

Management of early Parkinson disease should encompass a holistic approach to the patient, including surveillance of motor and nonmotor symptoms, exercise, and communication between patient and health care provider. Although treatment may not be indicated for milder symptoms, there is no reason for patients to endure present disability in order to hold off from medications for future use. It is hoped that, with the help of more advanced biomarkers, earlier diagnosis of Parkinson disease and medication management that is both neuroprotective and neurorestorative will be the future.

REFERENCES

1. Jankovic J. Parkinson's disease: clinical features and diagnosis. J Neurol Neurosurg Psychiatry 2008;79(4):368–76.
2. Hristova AH, Koller WC. Early Parkinson's disease: what is the best approach to treatment. Drugs Aging 2000;17(3):165–81.
3. Postuma RB, Berg D, Adler CH, et al. The new definition and diagnostic criteria of Parkinson's disease. Lancet Neurol 2016;15(6):546–8.
4. Collony BS, Lang AE. Pharmalogical treatment of Parkinson disease. JAMA 2014; 311(16):1670–83.
5. Carlsson A, Lindqvist M, Magnusson T. 3,4-Dihydroxyphenylala-nine and 5-hydroxytryptophan as reserpine antagonists. Nature 1957;180:1200.
6. Cotzias GC, Papavasiliou PS, Gellene R. Modification of Parkinsonism:chron ic treatme nt with L-dop a. N Engl J Med 1969;280:337–45.
7. Ovallath S, Sulthana B. Levodopa: history and therapeutic applications. Ann Indian Acad Neurol 2017;20(3):185–9.
8. Martin WE. Adverse reactions during treatment of Parkinson's disease with levodopa. JAMA 1971;216(12):1979–83.
9. Davie CA. A review of Parkinson's disease. Br Med Bull 2008;86:109–27.

10. Brooks JB. Dopamine agonists: their role in the treatment of Parkinson's disease. J Neurol Neurosurg Psychiatry 2000;68:685–9.
11. Stocchi F, Vacca L, Radicati FG. How to optimize the treatment of early stage Parkinson's disease. Transl Neurodegener 2015;4(4). https://doi.org/10.1186/2047-9158-4-4.
12. Riederer P, Laux G. MAO-inhibitors in Parkinson's disease. Exp Neurobiol 2011; 20(1):1–17.
13. Lees AJ. Drugs for Parkinson's disease. J Neurol Neurosurg Psychiatry 2002;73: 607–10.
14. Aminoff MJ, Christine CW, Friedman JH, et al. Management of the hospitalized patient with Parkinson's disease: current state of the field and need for guidelines. Parkinsonism Relat Disord 2011;17(3):139–45.
15. Oertel WH, Wolters E, Sampaio C, et al. Pergolide versus levodopa monotherapy in early Parkinson's disease patients: the PELMOPET study. Mov Disord 2006;21: 343–53.
16. Parkinson Study Group. Pramipexole vs levodopa as initial treatment for Parkinson disease: a randomized controlled trial. JAMA 2000;284(15):1931–8.
17. Rascol O, Brooks DJ, Korczyn AD, et al. A five-year study of the incidence of dyskinesia in patients with early Parkinson's disease who were treated with ropinirole or levodopa. N Engl J Med 2000;342(20):1484–91.
18. Fahn S. A new look at levodopa based on the ELLDOPA study. J Neural Transm Suppl 2006;70(Suppl):419–26.
19. Cilia R, Akpalu A, Sarfo FS, et al. The modern pre-levodopa era of Parkinson's disease: insights into motor complications from sub-Saharan Africa. Brain 2014;137(Pt 10):2731–42.
20. Olanow CW. Levodopa: effect on cell death and the natural history of Parkinson's disease. Mov Disord 2015;30:37–44.
21. Duncan GW, Khoo TK, Yarnall AJ, et al. Health-related quality of life in early Parkinson's disease: the impact of nonmotor symptoms. Mov Disord 2014;29: 195–202.
22. Suarez-Cedeno G, Suescun J, Schiess MC. Earlier intervention with deep brain stimulation for Parkinson's. Parkinsons Dis 2017. https://doi.org/10.1155/2017/9358153.
23. Deuschl G, Schade-Brittinger C, Krack P, et al. A randomized trial of deep brain stimulation for Parkinson's disease. N Engl J Med 2006;355:896–908.
24. Shuepbach WWM, Rau J, Knudsen K, et al. Neurostimulation for Parkinson's disease with early motor complications. N Engl J Med 2013;368:610–22.
25. Mestre TA, Espay AJ, Marras C, et al. Subthalamic nucleus-deep brain stimulation for early motor complications in Parkinson's disease—the EARLYSTIM trial: early is not always better. Mov Disord 2014;29:1751–6.
26. Prodoehl J, Rafferty MR, David FJ, et al. Two-year exercise program improves physical function in Parkinson's disease: the PRET-PD randomized clinical trial. Neurorehabil Neural Repair 2015;29(2):112–22.
27. Ahlskog EJ. Aerobic exercise: evidence for a direct brain effect to slow Parkinson's disease progression. Mayo Clin Proc 2018;93(3):360–72.
28. Corcos DM, Robichaud JA, David FJ, et al. A two-year randomized controlled trial of progressive resistance exercise for Parkinson's disease. Mov Disord 2013; 28(9):1230–40.

Management of Motor Features in Advanced Parkinson Disease

Henry Moore, MD*, Danielle S. Shpiner, MD,
Corneliu C. Luca, MD, PhD

KEYWORDS

- Parkinson disease • Advanced Parkinson disease • Motor fluctuations • Dyskinesias
- Deep brain stimulation

KEY POINTS

- Advanced Parkinson disease (PD) is characterized by the presence of motor complications requiring medical treatment, significant disability despite levodopa therapy, presence of postural instability, or levodopa-refractory symptoms.
- The main treatment during advanced PD is carbidopa/levodopa.
- Treatment of motor complications includes multiple pharmacologic and nonpharmacologic strategies.
- Patients with motor complications that failed pharmacologic therapies should be evaluated for pump therapies and deep brain stimulation.
- Levodopa-refractory symptoms require mostly nonpharmacologic interventions.

INTRODUCTION

Advanced PD is characterized by at least one of the following conditions: (1) presence of problematic motor complications from levodopa, either fluctuations or dyskinesias; (2) disability that interferes with independence despite levodopa therapy; (3) loss of postural reflexes leading to gait imbalance and falls; (4) presence of freezing phenomenon that markedly interferes with walking; or (5) marked postural deformities.[1]

DEFINING FLUCTUATIONS AND DYSKINESIAS

After an average of 3 years on levodopa, due to progressive degeneration of the dopaminergic system, patients with PD may start experiencing a variety of motor

Disclosure Statement: Dr H. Moore has served as consultant for TEVA, US World Meds, and UCB. Dr D.S. Shpiner has nothing to disclose. Dr C.C. Luca has served as consultant for Medtronic, Abbott, Boston Scientific, and AbbVie.
Division of Parkinson Disease and Movement Disorders, Department of Neurology, University of Miami, Miller School of Medicine, 1120 Northwest 14th Street, 1342, Miami, FL 33136, USA
* Corresponding author.
E-mail address: hmoore@med.miami.edu

Clin Geriatr Med 36 (2020) 43–52
https://doi.org/10.1016/j.cger.2019.09.010
0749-0690/20/© 2019 Elsevier Inc. All rights reserved.

complications. These are grouped into 2 categories: fluctuations (OFF states) and dyskinesias.

OFF states are characterized by a return of parkinsonian symptoms and signs (bradykinesia, tremor, rigidity) despite levodopa treatment. In contrast, during ON states, the parkinsonian symptoms are well controlled. The temporal relationship between the OFF states and the dosing of levodopa is very important to defining these fluctuations (**Table 1**). Initially, OFF periods (time spent in the OFF state) are predictable and usually appear before the next levodopa dose, termed end-of-dose wearing-off. Predictable wearing-off and the presence of PD symptoms in the morning before the first dose of levodopa (morning akinesia) tend to be the earliest manifestations of motor fluctuations.[2] As PD progresses, the OFF periods may become unpredictable and occur at any time, unrelated to levodopa dosing.[3]

Involvement of the enteric nervous system by PD pathology may precede the dopaminergic degeneration by several years, leading to gastroparesis and constipation.[4,5] Gastroparesis causes a delay in the passage of an oral dose of levodopa from the stomach to its place of absorption (distal duodenum and proximal jejunum), which delays its onset of effect. In addition, high-protein and -fat meals may further reduce gastrointestinal motility, aggravating the problem.[6]

Table 1 Features of motor fluctuations and dyskinesias in temporal relationship to levodopa dosing	
Off state	
Predictable wearing off	Reemergence of PD symptoms before the next levodopa dose
Unpredictable, sudden off	Sudden return of parkinsonian symptoms, unrelated to levodopa timing
Beginning of dose worsening and end of dose rebound	Transient worsening of PD symptoms at the beginning of the dose or at the end of dose. Usually presents with tremor.
Dose failure, delayed or partial on response	A dose of levodopa with a delayed effect (delayed on) or partial/no effect (dose failure)
Weak response at end of day	Gradual reduction of levodopa effect as the day progresses
Response variation in relationship to meals	Reduction of levodopa effect after a high-protein meal
"OFF" freezing	A transient difficulty initiating or continuing a movement (eg, at initiation of gait, while crossing doorways, while turning, while approaching to a target, while getting close to an obstacle/crowd)
"OFF" dystonia	Usually painful sustained contractions of distal leg muscles provoking abnormal postures
On State	
Peak of dose dyskinesia	A combination of chorea, ballism, and dystonia during peak of dose of levodopa
Diphasic dyskinesia	A combination of chorea, ballism, and dystonia at the beginning of the dose or at the end of the dose. Usually affects lower extremities, dystonic, stereotypic kicking
Myoclonus	Less frequent. Usually emerges within 10–20 min of a levodopa dose and tends to disappear in the fully on state
Respiratory dyskinesia	Irregular breath and rate of breathing because of involvement of respiratory muscles in peak-dose dyskinesia

Levodopa absorption may be affected by multiple factors. Large neutral amino acids, such as the ones contained in high-protein meals, compete with levodopa for absorption both at the gastrointestinal level and in the brain.[7] In addition, low gastric PH and other more controversial factors, including the presence of *Helicobacter pylori* in the stomach[8] and bacterial overgrowth in the small intestine, may interfere with levodopa absorption and worsen fluctuations.[9] This delayed and at times complete lack of absorption after an oral dose of levodopa contribute to the emergence of delayed ON states and failed doses.

In addition to motor fluctuations, the clinician should be aware of the presence of nonmotor fluctuations, which are characterized by one or more neuropsychiatric, autonomic, and sensory symptoms due to fluctuations in levodopa plasma levels (**Table 2**). At times, they may be more disabling than motor fluctuations, but if recognized early, can usually be easily controlled by adjusting the levodopa dose.[10]

Dyskinesias are abnormal involuntary movements that emerge a few years after initiating levodopa therapy and occur in temporal relationship to the levodopa dose (see **Table 1**). The most common type is known as peak dose dyskinesias, as they emerge during the peak of levodopa plasma level. The most common types of peak dose dyskinesias are chorea, ballism, and dystonia.[11] On rare occasions, peak dose dyskinesias may affect respiratory muscles.[10] Less commonly, dyskinesias may appear when dopamine levels are reduced or absent. This category includes diphasic dyskinesias and OFF period dystonia.[10] Diphasic dyskinesias appear either at the beginning of levodopa dose (as levodopa plasma levels increase) or at the end of dose (as levels decrease). They tend to affect the legs and involve slow stereotypical alternating leg movements, ballistic kicking, dystonia, and abnormal gait.[12] OFF period dystonia also tends to affect the legs and is manifested by ankle inversion, toes flexion, or extension.[10]

The presence of levodopa-induced motor complications and dyskinesias increases with disease progression and is estimated at 10% per year after initiation of levodopa therapy.[13] Based on several epidemiologic studies, patients with younger age at disease onset, longer use of levodopa, and higher individual doses are at increased risk of developing motor complications.[13] Patients with late-onset PD tend to have a lower risk of developing dyskinesias, hence the rationale for using levodopa as initial therapy.

TREATMENT OF MOTOR FLUCTUATIONS ASSOCIATED WITH LEVODOPA TREATMENT

The main treatment strategy for motor fluctuations involves characterizing when and how the OFF periods occur. This information can then be used to adjust timing and

Table 2
Features of non-motor fluctuations in temporal relationship to levodopa dosing

Off state	
Psychiatric	Anxiety, depression, panic attacks, apathy, fatigue
Cognitive	Reduction in executive function, attention, verbal fluency
Sensory	Paresthesia, numbness, dysesthesia, pain, akathisia (inner restlessness)
Autonomic	Urinary disturbances, bloating, abdominal pain, drooling, drenching sweats, cold hands and feet, flushing, pallor, hyperthermia, shortness of breath (air hunger without alterations in oxygenation)
On State	
Neuropsychiatric	Euphoria, agitation, mania/hypomania, impulses, illusions, hallucinations, delusions

dosages of medications to improve control of the most bothersome symptoms. Medications may also be changed to longer-acting formulations or additional medications may be added to prolong the duration of therapeutic effect.

The first step in managing end-of-dose wearing OFF periods is altering the timing of levodopa such as dividing total daily dose of levodopa into smaller, more frequent dosages or adding additional administration times of the same dose, depending on patient needs.[6] If the patient is experiencing delayed ON or failed doses, particularly after doses taken at the same time as protein-rich meals, adjusting the timing of meals and medications such that each dose is taken on an empty stomach (at least 30 minutes before meals) may optimize the levodopa effect.[6]

If adjusting the timing of medication dosing is not effective in decreasing end-of-dose wearing off, an option is switching the patient to a longer-acting formulation of levodopa. Two options are commercially available: carbidopa/levodopa controlled-release (Sinemet CR) and carbidopa/levodopa extended-release capsules (Rytary). The former, initially developed in the 1980s, has been shown to be effective in prolonging the beneficial effects of levodopa but is associated with inconsistent absorption, poor or delayed response, and worsening of peak-dose dyskinesias.[14,15] The latter, developed more recently, is able to reduce motor fluctuations and maintain ON time without producing troublesome dyskinesias.[14–16]

If the abovementioned strategies are ineffective or long-acting levodopa formulations are cost prohibitive, another option is to add an additional agent. Dopamine agonists, which are also commonly used as monotherapy in mild to moderate PD, have been shown to prolong the effects of levodopa when used in combination.[17] They should be used with caution in elderly patients due to their side effect profile, which includes orthostatic hypotension, hallucinations, confusion, somnolence, lower extremity edema, and impulse control disorder.[15] Monoamine oxidase B inhibitors, such as selegiline (Eldepryl), rasagiline (Azilect), and Safinamide (Xadago), can be added in an attempt to extend the effects of levodopa. They act by inhibiting the metabolism of dopamine centrally.[18] Entacapone (Comtan), a catechol-O-methyltransferase inhibitor can be added to each dose of levodopa to block the metabolism of levodopa in the periphery, thereby enhancing its bioavailability in the central nervous system and extending the effect duration.[19] These drugs are effective in reducing OFF time; however, they also increase the risk of dyskinesias.[15]

Unpredictable OFF periods may at times improve with the above strategies; alternatively (or in combination), the clinician may consider adding a short-acting rescue therapy. There are 2 options currently on the market and another currently in clinical trials. The first is subcutaneous apomorphine, a rapidly acting dopamine agonist self-administered with an autoinjector device.[20] Onset of action is generally seen within 5 to 15 minutes, and effects last from 40 to 90 minutes.[21] The other is inhaled levodopa (Inbrija). This medication is administered by a capsule-based, breath-actuated passive inhaler.[22] In the largest phase III clinical trial evaluating its efficacy, improvement in motor symptoms was seen within 10 minutes after administration, and improvement in symptoms lasted for 1 hour.[22] A sublingual formulation of apomorphine is currently under investigation and may be another alternative in the future.[23]

Given the number of medications available for the treatment of PD with motor fluctuations, there are many different strategies that clinicians may try. Most movement disorder experts agree that all of the treatment options discussed earlier are effective, and if one is not sufficient, one or more alternatives can be tried and/or combined with greater success.[18]

Table 3 provides a summary of medications commonly used in the United States for the management of motor fluctuations.

Table 3
Summary of medications used for the treatment of motor fluctuations and dyskinesias

Medication Class	Commonly Used Examples (Brand Names)	Main Mechanism of Action	Use	Common Side Effects
Long-acting formulations of levodopa	Carbidopa/levodopa CR (Sinemet CR) Carbidopa/levodopa ER (Rytary)	Dopamine precursor	Control of motor symptoms; prolonged duration of effect compared with immediate release formulation	Nausea, orthostatic hypotension, dyskinesia, hallucinations
Dopamine agonists	Pramipexole (Mirapex) Ropinirole (Requip) Rotigotine (Neupro) patch	Agonists to dopamine receptor in CNS, potentiate effects of levodopa when used in combination	Alternative to levodopa in mild-moderate PD; used in combination with levodopa to prolong ON time	Somnolence, confusion, hallucinations, orthostatic hypotension, lower extremity edema, impulse control disorders
MAO-B inhibitors	Selegiline (Eldepryl) Rasagiline (Azilect) Safinamide (Xadago)	Inhibits levodopa metabolism in the CNS	Alternative to levodopa in mild-moderate PD; used in combination with levodopa to prolong ON time	Exacerbation of levodopa-induced effects
COMT inhibitors	Entacapone (Comtan) Carbidopa/levodopa/entacapone combination (Stalevo) Tolcapone (Tasmar)	Inhibits levodopa metabolism in the periphery	Used in combination with levodopa to prolong ON time	Dark-colored urine, exacerbation of levodopa-induced effects (entacapone); hepatotoxicity (tolcapone)
Rescue medications	Sublingual apomorphine (Apokyn) Inhaled levodopa (Inbrija)	Dopamine agonist (apomorphine); dopamine precursor (levodopa)	Used during sudden or unpredictable OFF time to help control symptoms until next scheduled dose of oral medication	Injection site reactions, other side effects similar to other dopamine agonists (apomorphine); cough, discolored mucus, nausea (inhaled levodopa)
NMDA antagonists	Amantadine (Symmetrel) Amantadine XR (Gocovri) Amantadine ER (Osmolex)	NMDA-receptor antagonist, potentiates dopamine release	Treatment of tremor and bradykinesia in mild-moderate PD; used to treat levodopa-induced dyskinesias	Hallucinations, confusion, blurry vision, nausea, dry mouth, constipation, livedo reticularis, lower extremity edema
Atypical antipsychotics	Clozapine (Clozaril)	D2 and 5-HT$_{2A}$ receptor antagonists	Treatment of levodopa-induced dyskinesias and PD psychosis	Agranulocytosis, myocarditis, seizures, sedation, orthostatic hypotension

Abbreviations: 5-HT$_{2A}$, serotonin type 2A; CNS, central nervous system; COMT, catechol-O-methyltransferase; CR, controlled release; D2, dopamine type 2; ER, extended release; MAO-B, monoamine oxidase type B; NMDA, N-methyl-D-aspartate.

TREATMENT OF DYSKINESIAS ASSOCIATED WITH LEVODOPA TREATMENT

The primary goal in managing patients with PD who have developed motor fluctuations is to reduce OFF time without causing or worsening bothersome dyskinesias.

Mild dyskinesias do not require treatment unless they become embarrassing for the patient or start to interfere with his or her daily life.[6,18] In fact, patients often prefer to be in the ON state with some dyskinesias, rather than OFF without them.[6] If the dyskinesias become bothersome, the first step in treatment involves reducing the doses of dopaminergic medications. If the patient is not able to tolerate doses low enough to control the dyskinesias, the next step would be to add an antidyskinesia agent. Amantadine is currently the most effective medication on the market for peak-dose dyskinesias and is available in both short-acting and long-acting formulations.[6,24] Clozapine is another option but is used less frequently due to the potential side effect of agranulocytosis and need for frequent blood monitoring.[19] Diphasic or off-period dyskinesias are treated by avoiding or minimizing OFF time and increasing dopamine levels as discussed in section III.[6]

Dyskinesias represent a common side effect of levodopa that is frequently feared by patients (and sometimes physicians). However, when they do occur, dyskinesias are usually not disabling and often not even noticeable to patients. When bothersome, there are several treatment options available to help minimize their effects on quality of life (see **Table 3**).

ADVANCED TREATMENTS OF PARKINSON DISEASE

As the disease progresses, motor fluctuations and dyskinesias may become more difficult to manage despite dose adjustments, formulation changes, addition of adjunct treatments, and rescue medications. In order to provide more ON time, decrease medication burden, and improve quality of life, several advanced treatment strategies can be considered. These include deep brain stimulation (DBS), levodopa-carbidopa intestinal gel infusion (LCIG), and subcutaneous infusion of apomorphine.

Deep Brain Stimulation

DBS is a well-established procedure that consists of delivery of continuous electrical impulses in the basal ganglia (subthalamic nucleus or internal globus pallidus) via implanted electrodes and an implantable generator, akin to a cardiac pacemaker. DBS is indicated for patients with PD with disease duration of more than 5 years and either motor complications that are not well-controlled with medications or tremor refractory to levodopa. Ideal DBS candidates are in good general health and still have a good response to levodopa punctuated by problematic OFF time or dyskinesias despite optimal medical therapy. Poor candidates include those who are no longer having a beneficial response to levodopa, those with severe impairment of gait and balance unrelated to motor fluctuations, significant cognitive impairment, atypical parkinsonism, untreated depression, or unrealistic expectations for the surgery.

Multiple randomized clinical trials have shown a significant improvement in motor symptoms, reduction in the total daily OFF time, and concomitant increase in ON time in patients with advanced PD post-DBS.[25,26] In the VA study, the ON time without troubling dyskinesia in the DBS group improved by a mean of 4.6 hours per day versus zero hours per day for the best medical therapy group.[26] Also, the total daily levodopa dose required to control the participants' symptoms was reduced significantly, and quality of life improved.

A common misconception among practitioners is that DBS is reserved as a last resort therapy and therefore patients are considered for the surgery in late stages of disease when balance and cognitive issues are the main problems. Although DBS is very effective in treating tremors, rigidity, and bradykinesia, it has no effects on postural stability or cognition and sometimes may worsen verbal fluency. Moreover, older patients are more likely to have complications postoperatively, such as confusion and urinary retention. The potential adverse effects of DBS are mostly related to the surgical procedure and implanted hardware; they include infection, intracerebral bleeding, stroke, weight gain, lead migration, and stimulation-related side effects.[25,26]

DBS effects are long-lasting and multiple studies have documented long-term outcomes. A meta-analysis examining outcomes at 4.5 years postsurgery showed sustained benefit in tremor, bradykinesia, and dyskinesia after DBS, whereas postural instability and gait dysfunction worsened despite some initial improvement.[27]

Levodopa-Carbidopa Intrajejunal Gel Infusion

The rationale behind the LCIG is the ability to reduce fluctuations in the levodopa serum levels and therefore achieve a more physiologic stimulation of dopamine receptors. By avoiding the pulsatile dopaminergic stimulation that occurs with oral levodopa, one can avoid OFF time and achieve continuous symptom control. The infusion is given continuously via a percutaneous endoscopic gastrostomy-jejunostomy feeding tube (PEG-J tube) with a portable infusion pump, usually with a morning dose followed by a continuous infusion over the course of 16 hours in patients with OFF time and motor fluctuations that are not controlled with oral medications. Patients who undergo the procedure experience a significant increase in ON time without dyskinesias and an overall improvement in quality of life.

Randomized clinical trials showed that LCIG is a viable alternative to DBS and an option for those unsuitable for surgery. In the pivotal trial that led to Food and Drug Administration (FDA) approval, the mean OFF time decreased by 4.04 hours for LCIG group compared with 2.14 hours in patients allocated to immediate-release oral levodopa-carbidopa.[28]

Serious potential adverse events include those related to the procedure (eg, pancreatitis, peritonitis), tube (kinking, displacement, need for replacement), or infusion system (mechanical problems, human factor issues), as well as the inconvenience of a pump system, increased risk of suicide, and polyneuropathy.[28] In a 12-month open-label study involving 298 patients with PD using LCIG, there were 2 serious adverse events of suicide, both in subjects younger than 65 years with a medical history of depression.[29] The investigators postulate that this higher risk of suicide may be related to the higher risk of depression in the advanced PD population rather than LCIG itself.[29] Physicians should be vigilant about the emotional state of all patients with advanced PD using LCIG infusion.

Subcutaneous Apomorphine Infusion

Apomorphine is a potent short-acting dopamine agonist that can be administered not only as a rescue therapy for OFF periods but also as a subcutaneous continuous infusion. The infusion formulation is under review by the FDA and has been used in several European countries. It is highly effective for reducing dyskinesias and the need for oral levodopa in patients with severe motor complications. A randomized double-blind trial to investigate the efficacy, safety, and tolerability of subcutaneous apomorphine infusion over a 12-week period showed that the apomorphine infusion significantly reduced OFF time compared with placebo. The main side effects were development of skin nodules in the injection sites, as well as somnolence, nausea, vomiting, confusion, visual hallucinations, and orthostatic hypotension.[30]

MRI-Guided Focused Ultrasound

Focused ultrasound is a minimally invasive technology that has been recently FDA approved for patients with refractory essential tremor and is being considered for patients with PD as well. The procedure produces a thermal lesion in the brain with the help of sonication delivered precisely in the target area under MRI guidance. Unilateral focused ultrasound subthalamotomy for the treatment of PD and pallidotomy for the treatment of levodopa-induced dyskinesias and cardinal motor symptoms of PD are currently under investigation.[31,32]

MANAGEMENT OF MOTOR SYMPTOMS REFRACTORY TO DOPAMINERGIC THERAPY

Many years after PD onset, the disease starts affecting structures outside the dopaminergic system including the brainstem and cerebral cortex, and as a result, certain motor symptoms in advanced PD are often resistant to dopaminergic medications.[6]

Falls are common and usually multifactorial. Common causes include postural instability (as demonstrated with an abnormal pull test), shuffling of gait (with short steps), festination (acceleration of gait speed with inability to stop), and/or freezing of gait. Freezing of gait can occur at gait initiation, or while crossing doorways, approaching a crowd, turning, and/or arriving at a destination. These symptoms may respond to higher doses of dopaminergic agents but are often refractory to medications. Factors associated with falls include orthopedic comorbidities, postural deformities, cognitive decline, and orthostatic hypotension. Physical therapy is key to assess the cause of falls and provide treatment. Patients with postural instability may benefit from waking aids (canes, walkers). Patients with freezing may benefit from floor cues (walking over a line on the floor or over caregiver's foot) and increasing turning space.[33]

Postural deformities affecting the axial skeleton can be present in advanced PD[34] and may include stooped posture, camptocormia (excessive flexion of the thoracolumbar spine while walking, which improves with sitting or lying supine), Pisa syndrome (lateral flexion of the spine), and head drop (forward flexion of cervical spine).[6] The cause is unclear but may be due to abnormal postural reflexes, dystonic mechanisms, and/or focal myopathy. Postural deformities typically do not respond to medications but may benefit from physical therapy and orthotic devices.[6] Botulinum toxin injections in the abdominal and lumbar spinal flexors and DBS have been beneficial in some patients with camptocormia; however, the evidence is limited and mostly coming from case reports and small open-label studies.[35]

Speech impairments worsen with advancing PD and include low volume (hypophonia), loss of prosody (monotone), and occasional bursts of rapid unintelligible speech (tachyphemia). Speech therapy (Lee Silverman Voice Treatment—LSVT LOUD), reading out loud, and singing may be beneficial.[36]

Refractory tremor can be present at any stage of the disease and may become disabling. Levodopa at high doses may help, but if there is no response, DBS may be beneficial.

SUMMARY

Treatment of patients with advanced PD is challenging. Levodopa remains the gold standard of treatment. Symptoms refractory to dopaminergic medications/levodopa are difficult to manage and may require the use of nonpharmacologic strategies.

REFERENCES

1. Fahn S. Medical treatment of Parkinson's disease. In: Fahn S, Jankovic J, editors. Principles and practice of movement disorders. 1st edition. London: Churchill Livingstone; 2007. p. 146–65.
2. Marsden CD, Parkes JD. "On-off" effects in patients with Parkinson's disease on chronic levodopa therapy. Lancet 1976;1(7954):292–6.
3. Fahn S. "On-off" phenomenon with levodopa therapy in Parkinsonism. Clinical and pharmacologic correlations and the effect of intramuscular pyridoxine. Neurology 1974;24(5):431–41.
4. Fasano A, Visanji NP, Liu LW, et al. Gastrointestinal dysfunction in Parkinson's disease. Lancet Neurol 2015;14(6):625–39.
5. Hawkes CH, Del Tredici K, Braak H. A timeline for Parkinson's disease. Parkinsonism Relat Disord 2010;16(2):79–84.
6. Morgan JC, Fox SH. Treating the motor symptoms of Parkinson disease. Continuum (Minneap Minn) 2016;22(4 Movement Disorders):1064–85.
7. Nutt JG, Carter JH, Lea ES, et al. Motor fluctuations during continuous levodopa infusions in patients with Parkinson's disease. Mov Disord 1997;12(3):285–92.
8. Rahne KE, Tagesson C, Nyholm D. Motor fluctuations and helicobacter pylori in Parkinson's disease. J Neurol 2013;260(12):2974–80.
9. Fasano A, Bove F, Gabrielli M, et al. The role of small intestinal bacterial overgrowth in Parkinson's disease. Mov Disord 2013;28(9):1241–9.
10. Aquino CC, Fox SH. Clinical spectrum of levodopa-induced complications. Mov Disord 2015;30(1):80–9.
11. Nutt JG. Levodopa-induced dyskinesia: review, observations, and speculations. Neurology 1990;40(2):340–5.
12. Luquin MR, Scipioni O, Vaamonde J, et al. Levodopa-induced dyskinesias in Parkinson's disease: clinical and pharmacological classification. Mov Disord 1992; 7(2):117–24.
13. Ahlskog JE, Muenter MD. Frequency of levodopa-related dyskinesias and motor fluctuations as estimated from the cumulative literature. Mov Disord 2001;16(3): 448–58.
14. LeWitt PA, Fahn S. Levodopa therapy for Parkinson disease: a look backward and forward. Neurology 2016;86(14 Suppl 1):S3–12.
15. Tarakad A, Jankovic J. Diagnosis and management of Parkinson's disease. Semin Neurol 2017;37(2):118–26.
16. Pahwa R, Lyons KE, Hauser RA, et al. Randomized trial of IPX066, carbidopa/levodopa extended release, in early Parkinson's disease. Parkinsonism Relat Disord 2014;20(2):142–8.
17. Oertel W, Schulz JB. Current and experimental treatments of Parkinson disease: a guide for neuroscientists. J Neurochem 2016;139(Suppl 1):325–37.
18. Connolly BS, Lang AE. Pharmacological treatment of Parkinson disease: a review. JAMA 2014;311(16):1670–83.
19. Fox SH, Katzenschlager R, Lim SY, et al. The movement disorder society evidence-based medicine review update: treatments for the motor symptoms of parkinson's disease. Mov Disord 2011;26(Suppl 3):S2–41.
20. Boyle A, Ondo W. Role of apomorphine in the treatment of Parkinson's disease. CNS Drugs 2015;29(2):83–9.
21. Stacy M, Silver D. Apomorphine for the acute treatment of "off" episodes in Parkinson's disease. Parkinsonism Relat Disord 2008;14(2):85–92.

22. LeWitt PA, Hauser RA, Pahwa R, et al. Safety and efficacy of CVT-301 (levodopa inhalation powder) on motor function during off periods in patients with Parkinson's disease: a randomised, double-blind, placebo-controlled phase 3 trial. Lancet Neurol 2019;18(2):145–54.

23. Hauser RA, Olanow CW, Dzyngel B, et al. Sublingual apomorphine (APL-130277) for the acute conversion of OFF to ON in Parkinson's disease. Mov Disord 2016; 31(9):1366–72.

24. da Silva-Junior FP, Braga-Neto P, Sueli Monte F, et al. Amantadine reduces the duration of levodopa-induced dyskinesia: a randomized, double-blind, placebo-controlled study. Parkinsonism Relat Disord 2005;11(7):449–52.

25. Deuschl G, Schade-Brittinger C, Krack P, et al. A randomized trial of deep-brain stimulation for Parkinson's disease. N Engl J Med 2006;355(9):896–908.

26. Weaver FM, Follett K, Stern M, et al. Bilateral deep brain stimulation vs best medical therapy for patients with advanced Parkinson disease: a randomized controlled trial. JAMA 2009;301(1):63–73.

27. St George RJ, Nutt JG, Burchiel KJ, et al. A meta-regression of the long-term effects of deep brain stimulation on balance and gait in PD. Neurology 2010;75(14): 1292–9.

28. Olanow CW, Kieburtz K, Odin P, et al. Continuous intrajejunal infusion of levodopa-carbidopa intestinal gel for patients with advanced Parkinson's disease: a randomised, controlled, double-blind, double-dummy study. Lancet Neurol 2014;13(2):141–9.

29. Fernandez HH, Standaert DG, Hauser RA, et al. Levodopa-carbidopa intestinal gel in advanced Parkinson's disease: final 12-month, open-label results. Mov Disord 2015;30(4):500–9.

30. Katzenschlager R, Poewe W, Rascol O, et al. Apomorphine subcutaneous infusion in patients with Parkinson's disease with persistent motor fluctuations (TOLEDO): a multicentre, double-blind, randomised, placebo-controlled trial. Lancet Neurol 2018;17(9):749–59.

31. Martinez-Fernandez R, Rodriguez-Rojas R, Del Alamo M, et al. Focused ultrasound subthalamotomy in patients with asymmetric Parkinson's disease: a pilot study. Lancet Neurol 2018;17(1):54–63.

32. Na YC, Chang WS, Jung HH, et al. Unilateral magnetic resonance-guided focused ultrasound pallidotomy for Parkinson disease. Neurology 2015;85(6): 549–51.

33. Okuma Y. Practical approach to freezing of gait in Parkinson's disease. Pract Neurol 2014;14(4):222–30.

34. Doherty KM, van de Warrenburg BP, Peralta MC, et al. Postural deformities in Parkinson's disease. Lancet Neurol 2011;10(6):538–49.

35. Srivanitchapoom P, Hallett M. Camptocormia in Parkinson's disease: definition, epidemiology, pathogenesis and treatment modalities. J Neurol Neurosurg Psychiatry 2016;87(1):75–85.

36. Mahler LA, Ramig LO, Fox C. Evidence-based treatment of voice and speech disorders in Parkinson disease. Curr Opin Otolaryngol Head Neck Surg 2015;23(3): 209–15.

Orthostatic Hypotension in Parkinson Disease

Jose-Alberto Palma, MD, PhD, Horacio Kaufmann, MD*

KEYWORDS

- Autonomic failure • Baroreflex dysfunction • Droxidopa • Midodrine
- Norepinephrine • Neurogenic orthostatic hypotension

KEY POINTS

- Approximately 50% of patients with Parkinson disease have orthostatic hypotension, although it is symptomatic in only a third of these patients.
- Orthostatic hypotension in Parkinson disease is usually neurogenic, which is because of inappropriate release of norepinephrine from sympathetic terminals when standing.
- Diagnosis of orthostatic hypotension requires blood pressure measurements. A heart rate increase below 0.5 beat per minute for each mm Hg fall in systolic blood pressure (ie, $\Delta HR/\Delta SBP$ ratio below 0.5 bpm/mm Hg) has high sensitivity and specificity to diagnose neurogenic orthostatic hypotension.
- The goal of treatment of orthostatic hypotension is not to normalize standing blood pressure, but to reduce symptom burden to improve quality of life.
- The steps in management are correction of aggravating factors and implementation of nonpharmacologic measures and pharmacologic therapies, including fludrocortisone, midodrine, droxidopa, and norepinephrine reuptake inhibitors.

INTRODUCTION

Dysfunction of the autonomic nervous system is a characteristic feature of patients with Parkinson disease and other synucleinopathies, a group of neurodegenerative

Disclosures: Dr J-.A. Palma has served on advisory boards of Lunbeck and Biogen. Dr J-.A. Palma is the principal investigator in clinical trials for neurogenic orthostatic hypotension sponsored by Theravance. Dr J-.A. Palma is managing editor of *Clinical Autonomic Research*. Dr J-.A. Palma has received grant support from the National Institutes of Health (NIH), US Food and Drug Administration (FDA), Familial Dysautonomia Foundation, and Michael J. Fox Foundation. Dr H. Kaufmann has served on advisory boards of Lunbeck, Biogen, Biohaven, and Theravance. He has been principal investigator in clinical trials for neurogenic orthostatic hypotension sponsored by Chelsea and Theravance. Dr H. Kaufmann is editor-in-chief of *Clinical Autonomic Research*. Dr H. Kaufmann has received grant support from the NIH, FDA, Familial Dysautonomia Foundation, and Michael J. Fox Foundation.
Department of Neurology, Dysautonomia Center, New York University School of Medicine, NYU Langone Health, 530 First Avenue, Suite 9Q, New York, NY 10016, USA
* Corresponding author.
E-mail address: Horacio.Kaufmann@nyulangone.org

diseases caused by the abnormal accumulation of misfolded phosphorylated α-syn-uclein (αSyn) in neurons, glia, or both.

Converging evidence indicates that abnormal αSyn spreads from cell to cell in a prion-like fashion[1–3] and that different types of αSyn assemblies with different structural characteristics called strains[4,5] may account for the different clinical phenotypes, as they determine the nerve cell type and the regions of the nervous system that are affected.[4] In patients with Parkinson disease, dementia with Lewy bodies (DLB), and pure autonomic failure (PAF), aggregates of misfolded αSyn accumulate in the neuronal soma and throughout axons, called Lewy bodies (LBs) and Lewy neurites, and peripheral autonomic neurons are always affected. In these patients, neurodegeneration usually progresses slowly with only a minor impact on survival.[6] In patients with multiple system atrophy (MSA), a rare and devastating disease, αSyn accumulates primarily in oligodendroglia, although neurons are also affected.[7,8] Autonomic dysfunction in synucleinopathies occurs at all stages of the disease and occasionally is its only manifestation.[9]

Among the most debilitating manifestations of autonomic dysfunction in Parkinson disease is orthostatic hypotension (OH), which is a sustained fall in blood pressure (BP) on standing. The current definition of OH, based on expert consensus,[10] is a fall of at least 20 mm Hg in systolic BP or 10 mm Hg in diastolic BP within 3 minutes of standing or upright tilt. OH can impair perfusion to organs above the heart, most notably the brain, resulting in symptoms of tissue hypoperfusion. Symptoms can be disabling, have a profound impact on a patient's quality of life, and increase morbidity and mortality.[11,12]

In Parkinson disease and other synucleinopathies, OH is neurogenic (nOH), that is, caused by reduced norepinephrine release from postganglionic efferent sympathetic nerves, resulting in defective vasoconstriction when assuming the upright posture (Fig. 1).[10] Complicating nOH management is arterial hypertension when supine (SH), which occurs in up to 50% of patients with efferent baroreflex failure.[13,14] When recognized, nOH can be treated, sometimes successfully. Discontinuation of potentially causative/aggravating drugs, patient education, nonpharmacological approaches, and pathophysiology-based drug therapy are keys to an effective management.

This article reviews the epidemiology, evaluation, and management of nOH, with emphasis on patients with Parkinson disease; it also summarizes the nonpharmacologic and pharmacologic treatment strategies and provides practical advice on the management of patients with this debilitating condition.

EPIDEMIOLOGY

In cross-sectional studies, between 30% and 50% of patients with Parkinson disease have OH.[14–17] The prevalence of OH in Parkinson disease increases with age and disease duration.[14] Although the prevalence of nOH in Parkinson disease is relatively high, not all patients have symptoms of organ hypoperfusion and only a third of patients (approximately 16%) have symptomatic nOH.[14] Symptomatic nOH in Parkinson disease is typically associated with an upright mean BP below 75 mm Hg. This value (a standing mean BP <75 mm Hg) has a sensitivity of 97% and a specificity of 98% for detecting symptomatic nOH and appears to be the lower limit of cerebrovascular autoregulation in patients with Parkinson disease and nOH, below which patients develop symptoms of cerebral hypoperfusion. Patients fulfilling criteria for nOH who also have SH are less likely to develop symptomatic nOH after 3 minutes of standing.

PATHOPHYSIOLOGY

Normally, unloading of the baroreceptors by standing up triggers norepinephrine release from postganglionic sympathetic efferent nerves, causing vasoconstriction,

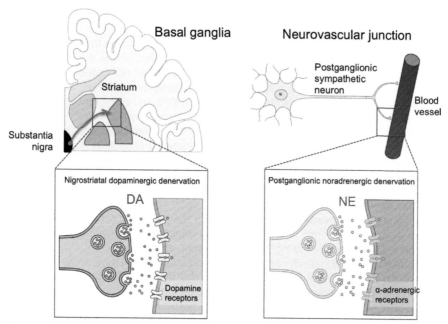

Fig. 1. Neurotransmitter disorders in Parkinson disease. Neurogenic orthostatic hypotension can be understood as a neurotransmitter disorder, similar to the motor dysfunction. Nigrostriatal dopaminergic denervation causing defective dopamine (DA) release results in the movement disorder, whereas postganglionic sympathetic denervation causing defective norepinephrine (NE) release when standing causes neurogenic orthostatic hypotension.

which maintains BP in the standing position. This compensatory vasoconstriction is absent or attenuated in patients with synucleinopathies, resulting in nOH. In patients with Parkinson disease, baroreflex dysfunction is predominantly caused by degeneration of postganglionic efferent sympathetic neurons. There is robust imaging and neuropathological data showing that postganglionic efferent sympathetic neurons innervating the myocardium are functionally affected because of αSyn deposits and fiber loss.[18,19] Sympathetic fibers innervating blood vessels are also affected. This results in impaired norepinephrine release and defective vasoconstriction upon standing, causing the BP to fall (ie, nOH).[16,19] Plasma norepinephrine, a marker of sympathetic neuronal integrity, is lower in patients with Parkinson disease and nOH than in those without nOH.[20]

APPROACH TO THE PATIENT WITH ORTHOSTATIC HYPOTENSION

OH can be symptomatic or asymptomatic. Typical symptoms of OH are lightheadedness, dizziness, blurry vision, and, when the fall in BP is pronounced, loss of consciousness and postural tone (syncope). Symptoms occur only when standing, less frequently when sitting, and abate when lying down. Patients with OH may also complain of generalized weakness, fatigue, leg buckling, occipital headache, neck and shoulder (coat hanger) discomfort, and shortness of breath caused by ventilation/perfusion mismatch in the apical lung areas.

Patients with chronic nOH caused by neurologic disorders usually tolerate very low BPs with only mild or no symptoms at all, but syncope can occur with added orthostatic stressors (eg, large carbohydrate-rich meals, alcohol intake, very warm weather, dehydration, and antihypertensive treatment).

Symptoms of OH typically disappear after the patient resumes the sitting or lying position, because cerebral blood flow is restored to levels above the lower limit of autoregulatory capacity (see **Fig. 1**). The chronic nature of nOH allows remarkable adaptive changes in cerebral autoregulatory mechanisms.[21] Indeed, patients with nOH are frequently able to tolerate wide swings in BPs and often remain conscious at pressures that would otherwise induce syncope in healthy subjects.[22]

Symptoms of nOH can be nonspecific, including fatigue and difficultly concentrating and may sometimes mimic a levodopa off motor state in PD patients. In these cases, the diagnosis of nOH may be missed unless BP is measured in the standing position. Conversely, it is important to realize that in patients with Parkinson disease, postural lightheadedness mimicking nOH may be caused by abnormal postural reflexes, vestibular deficits, or orthostatic tremor.[23]

In contrast to vasovagal (neurally mediated) syncope, syncope in nOH occurs without signs of autonomic activation such as diaphoresis, tachycardia, nausea, or abdominal discomfort. Following syncope, as soon as they resume the supine position, patients with nOH usually recover quickly and may be unaware of the event. Patients report that symptom severity varies from day to day and fluctuates throughout the day. The morning hours tend to be most difficult, as OH symptoms are aggravated by intravascular volume loss overnight.[24] Meals, particularly carbohydrate-rich meals, lead to splanchnic vasodilatation and postprandial hypotension (ie, fall in BP within 2 hours of eating). The severity of postprandial hypotension is directly related to insulin release.[25] This has therapeutic implications as will be later discussed. Physical inactivity and prolonged bed rest are common in patients with nOH. This leads to cardiovascular deconditioning, further worsening the fall in BP and increasing symptoms, leading to a vicious cycle.

Patients at high risk should be routinely screened for OH, even in the absence of symptoms. These include patients with a synucleinopathy (Parkinson disease/DLB, MSA, or PAF), elderly subjects (>70 year old), or patients on multiple medications.

DIAGNOSIS OF NEUROGENIC ORTHOSTATIC HYPOTENSION

In patients presenting with orthostatic intolerance (ie, difficulty maintaining the upright position), it is necessary to determine whether symptoms are caused by orthostatic hypotension or other causes (**Table 1**).

The diagnosis of OH requires BP readings while supine and upright, either during active standing or during a tilt-table test, to determine the presence of a sustained orthostatic fall of at least 20 mm Hg systolic or 10 mm Hg diastolic BP. BP and heart rate should be measured after the patient has been supine for several minutes and after standing still (or passively tilted) for 1 to 3 minutes. The magnitude of the BP fall and symptom severity varies at different times of the day; thus it may be necessary to retest the patient in the morning when the orthostatic fall in pressure is more pronounced or after a meal if the history suggests postprandial hypotension.

In patients reporting typical symptoms but without a fall in BP within 3 minutes of standing, a more prolonged orthostatic stress with a tilt-table test may be necessary to define the condition. Patients with milder or earlier forms of efferent baroreflex failure may experience orthostatic hypotension after longer time standing (ie, delayed orthostatic hypotension).[26,27] Patients may report symptoms mimicking those of orthostatic hypotension but without an identified fall in BP not infrequently, and these patients include those with vestibular disorders, gait abnormalities, reported use of

Table 1
Distinguishing features of neurogenic and non-neurogenic orthostatic hypotension

	Non-neurogenic Orthostatic Hypotension	Neurogenic Orthostatic Hypotension
Epidemiology	Typically elderly	Typically middle-aged
Onset	Variable	Usually chronic (acute or subacute with immune-mediated etiology)
Causes	Intravascular volume loss (eg, dehydration, anemia) Blood pooling (eg, large varicose veins, skeletal muscle atrophy) Advanced heart failure Adrenal insufficiency Physical deconditioning Antihypertensive medications	Reduced norepinephrine release from sympathetic posganglionic nerves when standing up
Prognosis	Resolves when underlying cause is corrected	Chronic disorder
Sympathetic tone	Increased	Low or absent
Increase in heart rate upon standing	Pronounced	Mild or absent
ΔHR/ΔSBP ratio	>0.5 bpm/mm Hg	<0.5 bpm/mm Hg
Blood pressure overshoot (phase 4) in Valsalva maneuver	Present	Absent
Increase in plasma norepinephrine levels upon standing	Normal or enhanced (at least x2)	Reduced or absent (less than x2)
Other symptoms of autonomic failure	No	Gastrointestinal dysfunction Urinary dysfunction Sudomotor abnormalities Erectile dysfunction (men)
Concomitant neurologic deficits	None (or if present, they are unrelated to orthostatic hypotension)	None Parkinsonism Cerebellar signs Cognitive impairment Sensory neuropathy

alcohol and drugs that depress the central nervous system (CNS), and inebriation-like syndrome.[23] Conversely, patients with cognitive impairment may not accurately identify symptoms of organ hypoperfusion, despite low BP when standing.[28]

If sustained orthostatic hypotension is confirmed, it is key to establish whether the cause is a pathologic lesion in sympathetic neurons (ie, neurogenic orthostatic hypotension) or if it is secondary to other medical causes (ie, non-neurogenic orthostatic hypotension) such as anemia- or dehydration-related volume depletion, excessive venous pooling sometimes aggravated by varicose veins, or medication adverse effects (eg, antihypertensive agents, diuretics, tricyclic antidepressants, opioids, benzodiazepines, and antiparkinsonian agents). Several features are useful to distinguish neurogenic versus non-neurogenic orthostatic hypotension (see **Table 1**). A heart rate increase of at least 0.5 beat per minute for each mm Hg fall in systolic blood pressure (ie, $\Delta HR/\Delta SBP$ ratio $\geq$0.5 bpm/mm Hg) has high sensitivity and specificity to diagnose non-neurogenic orthostatic hypotension. Conversely, a $\Delta HR/\Delta SBP$ ratio less than 0.5 bpm/mm Hg indicates neurogenic orthostatic hypotension.[29]

Ambulatory BP monitoring (ABPM) can assist in the diagnosis and management of nOH.[30] Affected patients typically have a reversal of the normal circadian BP pattern, with higher BP during the night when the patient is supine in bed than during the day. Nocturnal SH causes pressure natriuresis with exaggerated sodium and water loss, causing overnight depletion of intravascular volume, worsening OH in the morning. ABPM and a detailed diary of activities are also useful to specifically tailor the use of short-acting pressor agents only at times when OH is severe in patients who may remain seated for long periods of the day or are wheelchair-bound.

MANAGEMENT OF NEUROGENIC ORTHOSTATIC HYPOTENSION

The goal of treatment is not to normalize standing BP, but to reduce symptom burden and improve quality of life. Consensus guidelines for the treatment of nOH are currently lacking, and there are no long-term studies analyzing the impact of treatment on survival, falls, or quality of life.

A noteworthy percentage of patients with nOH also have SH, which poses a difficult therapeutic challenge. In a multicenter study including 210 patients with PD from the United States and Europe, 44% had a supine BP greater than140/90 mm Hg.[14] Similar results (45% prevalence of SH) were found in a sample of 72 patients with PD from Japan.[31] Another study found that 71% of patients with PD had absent or reversed nocturnal BP dipping, as measured by ABPM, which is another way of quantifying SH.[13]

Drugs that can increase BP while in the upright position can worsen SH. Therefore, pharmacologic treatment of nOH requires careful consideration of the potential risks and actual benefits.

The steps in management include: correcting aggravating factors, implementing nonpharmacological measures, and drug therapies.

Correction of Aggravating Factors

Drugs that reduce intravascular volume (diuretics), induce vasodilatation (sildenafil, nitrates), or block norepinephrine release/activity at the neurovascular junction (α-blockers, centrally acting α_2-agonists, and tricyclic antidepressants) worsen nOH and symptoms. Levodopa and dopamine agonists may also lower BP, and a dose adjustment may be considered based on an individual risk-benefit assessment.[32–35] Anemia should be investigated and treated.[36] Erythropoietin (25–50 units/kg, subcutaneous, 3 times a week) in conjunction with iron supplements may be beneficial in patients with nOH and anemia.[37]

Nonpharmacologic Treatment and Patient Education

Nonpharmacologic measures are summarized in **Box 1**. Patients should be aware of the diuretic effects of caffeine and alcohol and avoid sugary beverages (eg, bottled juices or sodas) because of the hypotensive effects of high-glycemic index carbohydrates.[25] Fluid intake should be 2 to 2.5 L/d. Patients should be encouraged to increase salt intake by adding 1 to 2 teaspoon of salt to a healthy diet. Other patients prefer using 0.5 to 1.0 g salt tablets, although they can cause abdominal discomfort. In patients with nOH, drinking 0.5 L of water produces a marked increase in BP.[38] This can be used as a rescue measure, because the pressor effect is quick (peaks in around 30 minutes), although short-lived.

Box 1
Nonpharmacological treatments for orthostatic hypotension

- Liberalization of salt consumption
- Liberalization of water intake (up to 2.5 L/d)
- Acute water bolus (drinking 500 mL of water)
- Sleeping with the head of the bed raised 30° to 45° with the help of an electric bed or mattress
- Physical activity with recumbent exercises (eg, stationary bicycle, or rowing machine) or in a swimming pool
- Physical countermaneuvers (eg, standing up slowly, leg crossing, or buttock clenching)[49]
- Abdominal binder[51]
- Compression waist-high stockings producing at least 15 to 20 mm Hg pressure[50] (knee- or thigh-high stockings are typically not useful)

Symptomatic nOH can quickly lead to a reluctance to stand up and avoidance of physical activity. In turn, physical immobility worsens OH, leading to a vicious cycle of deconditioning.[11] Physical exercise is therefore a key component of the therapeutic regimen, but because physical activity in the standing position can worsen hypotension in patients with efferent baroreflex failure,[39–42] exercise should be performed in the recumbent or sitting position using a recumbent stationary bicycle or rowing machine. The exception is exercise in a pool, as the hydrostatic pressure of water allows upright exercise without hypotension.[43] Patients should be taught specific physical countermaneuvers.[44] Eating results in blood pooling within the splanchnic circulation, and patients can become severely hypotensive within 2 hours of eating (ie, postprandial hypotension), particularly after carbohydrate-rich meals.[10,45–47] Eating smaller, more frequent meals and reducing carbohydrates can improve postprandial hypotension. Alcohol is also a vasodilator and should be reserved for the evening, prior to going to bed.

Patients should be instructed to change positions gradually, and briefly sit before standing. Straining and Valsalva-like maneuvers during bowel movements are a common cause of syncope.[48] If this is the case, constipation must be treated aggressively.[49] High-waist compression stockings producing at least 15–20 mm Hg of pressure can increase BP by augmenting venous return.[50] Patients with movement disorders struggle to put the stockings on, which limits their usefulness in everyday life. Elastic abdominal binders are a good alternative.[51,52] A recently developed abdominal binder that inflates automatically only on standing has shown promising results in patients with nOH.[53]

Pharmacologic management

Although nonpharmacologic methods are effective when performed properly, many patients with nOH still require pharmacologic treatment to improve symptoms. Two complementary strategies are used: expanding intravascular volume with the synthetic mineralocorticoid fludrocortisone and increasing peripheral vascular resistance with the pressor agents midodrine or droxidopa. Selection of one or the other or both depends on the specific features and needs of each patient. Fludrocortisone can be combined with midodrine or droxidopa. No studies have directly compared midodrine and droxidopa, so whether 1 method exerts more symptomatic relief than the other is unknown.

All available drugs that raise BP in the standing position also raise BP in the supine position, therefore increasing the risk or worsening SH. Although there are no specific data on cardiovascular and cerebrovascular events induced by SH in patients with nOH, treating physicians should be aware of this potential adverse effect. Before beginning treatment with fludrocortisone, midodrine, or droxidopa, the patient's medication should be carefully reviewed.

Combination therapy of agents that increase BP (eg, fludrocortisone, ephedrine, midodrine, droxidopa, and triptans) increases the risk of SH.

Patients should be instructed to avoid the supine position during the day, to sleep with the head of the bed raised 30°, and to ensure that they take their final dose of droxidopa or midodrine at least 4 hours before bedtime. Droxidopa or midodrine should be reduced, and, if necessary, discontinued if severe SH persists. BP should be rechecked supine at a 30° angle if increased doses are required. Safety in patients with BP higher than 180 mm Hg at a 30° angle has not been established, as these patients were excluded from the clinical trials that led to drug approval.

Fludrocortisone Fludrocortisone (9α-fluorocortisol) is a synthetic mineralocorticoid that increases renal sodium and water reabsorption, therefore expanding intravascular volume and increasing BP in all positions. Experimental data suggest that fludrocortisone enhances the pressor effect of norepinephrine and angiotensin II. Although not specifically approved by the US Food and Drug Administration (FDA) for this indication, fludrocortisone is perhaps the most frequently prescribed agent for the treatment of orthostatic hypotension. Because activation of renal mineralocorticoid receptors results in inflammation and fibrosis and may have a direct nephrotoxic effect leading to a faster decline in renal function and hypertension,[54] fludrocortisone should be used with extreme caution in the treatment of orthostatic hypotension, preferably for short-term periods, and dosage should never be higher than 0.2 mg/d. Higher dosages do not have improved therapeutic effects but do intensify adverse effects. Fludrocortisone usually requires at least 7 to 10 days of treatment to exert any significant clinical effect. Short-term adverse effects are frequent and include supine hypertension, hypokalemia, and ankle edema.[55] To reduce the risk of hypokalemia, patients taking fludrocortisone should be instructed to eat potassium-rich foods or to take potassium supplements (potassium chloride 20 mEq a day). Long-term use exacerbates permanent hypertension and target damage,[54] including left ventricular hypertrophy[56] and renal failure[54] and is associated with a higher risk of all-cause hospitalization in patients with orthostatic hypotension.[57]

Midodrine Midodrine is an oral α_1-adrenoceptor agonist that induces vasoconstriction and increases BP.[58–61] Midodrine is approved for the treatment of symptomatic OH in the United States, Europe, and Asia. Midodrine raises BP in the standing, sitting, and supine positions, and its pressor effect is noticeable approximately 30 to 45 minutes after consumption, reaching a maximum after approximately 1 hour, and persists for a total of 2 to 3 hours. Treatment should begin with a 2.5 or 5 mg dose, which can then be increased up to 10 mg to be taken up to 3 times a day. nSH is common; hence, patients should not take midodrine less than 3 to 4 hours before bedtime. Other adverse events owing to activation of α1-adrenergic receptors are piloerection (goosebumps), itching of the scalp, and urinary retention. Midodrine has no effect on heart rate, as it does not activate β-adrenoreceptors, and, given its poor diffusion across the blood-brain barrier, has no CNS adverse effects.[62]

Droxidopa Droxidopa (L-threo-3,4-dihydroxyphenyl-serine, L-DOPS) is an oral synthetic amino acid that is converted to norepinephrine in the body.[63] Droxidopa is decarboxylated to norepinephrine by the enzyme aromatic amino acid decarboxylase (AAAD), the same enzyme the converts L-dopa to dopamine. Droxidopa was approved in Japan in 1989 for the treatment of nOH in PD, MSA, and familial amyloid polyneuropathy. In the United States, the FDA approved droxidopa in 2014 for the treatment of symptomatic nOH associated with PAF, Parkinson disease, and MSA.[64–68] Droxidopa is not approved in Europe. Extensive clinical experience shows that droxidopa is safe and well tolerated.[69–77] Peak plasma concentrations of droxidopa are reached approximately 3 hours after oral administration. The dosage used in clinical trials was 100 to 600 mg 3 times daily, although clinical experience indicates that the dosage should be tailored to each patient's needs, considering the periods of time when he or she is going to be active or inactive.[63,70,75] Because the pressor effect of droxidopa varies among patients, a titration procedure supervised by a clinician is highly recommended.[16] Ambulatory 24-h BP monitoring (ABPM) is useful to evaluate the BP profile before and after initiating treatment with droxidopa.[78]

Inhibition of the AAAD with high doses of carbidopa can abolish the pressor effect of droxidopa by preventing its peripheral conversion to norepinephrine. This was shown in studies using a single 200 mg dose of carbidopa administered 30 minutes before droxidopa.[79] In clinical practice, the dose of carbidopa in patients treated with L-dopa is lower than 200 mg; thus carbidopa appears not to block the pressor effect of droxidopa significantly.[69] Further studies are warranted to determine whether droxidopa has beneficial effects on other motor and nonmotor symptoms that result from norepinephrine deficiency in patients with PD.[80]

Norepinephrine reuptake inhibitors An emerging approach in the treatment of neurogenic orthostatic hypotension is the use of inhibitors of the norepinephrine membrane transporter, which inhibit norepinephrine reuptake and increase its availability in the neurovascular junction.

In healthy subjects, norepinephrine reuptake inhibition has little effect on blood pressure. The reason is that, although norepinephrine reuptake inhibitors enhance noradrenergic vasoconstriction at the level of the sympathetic postganglionic fibers, this is counteracted by norepinephrine-mediated central α_2-receptors stimulation in the CNS, which has a vasodilator effect. However, in patients with central autonomic dysfunction, norepinephrine reuptake inhibitors result in only peripheral vasoconstriction, making this therapeutic group particularly suitable for patients with MSA.

Short-term controlled clinical trials have shown that atomoxetine (10–18 mg, twice a day), a short-acting norepinephrine reuptake inhibitor, increases standing BP and reduces the burden of symptoms compared to placebo in patients with neurogenic orthostatic hypotension.[81–83] The higher the norepinephrine levels, the greater the pressor effect and symptomatic improvement with atomoxetine, which makes it a particularly attractive option for patients with neurogenic orthostatic hypotension caused by autonomic decentralization (eg, MSA).[84] A multicenter controlled trial to confirm the efficacy of atomoxetine in patients with neurogenic orthostatic hypotension is underway (ClinicalTrials.gov NCT02784535). A phase 2 trial with ampreloxetine (TD-9855), a long-acting investigational norepinephrine reuptake inhibitor, showed that this compound was safe and increased BP and orthostatic tolerance in patients with neurogenic orthostatic hypotension; a large multicenter phase 3 study to confirm this is ongoing (ClinicalTrials.gov NCT03750552).

Conversely, lower supine plasma norepinephrine levels appear to predict a greater symptomatic and pressor response to droxidopa, a synthetic oral norepinephrine precursor.[85] These responses can be explained by denervation supersensitivity of adrenergic receptors.[86] Consequently, patients with low plasma norepinephrine levels (usually LB disorders or peripheral autonomic neuropathies) may respond better to droxidopa and midodrine,[85] whereas patients with normal or high norepinephrine levels (usually MSA) may respond better to norepinephrine reuptake inhibitors.

In patients with refractory neurogenic orthostatic hypotension, norepinephrine reuptake inhibition could be theoretically combined with droxidopa or midodrine, with or without fludrocortisone or pyridostigmine. However, no safety data are available on the combined use of most of these agents, and extreme caution is advised.

Other medications Pyridostigmine, an inhibitor of cholinesterase, the enzyme that catalyzes the hydrolysis of acetylcholine and terminates its action, potentiates cholinergic neurotransmission in autonomic ganglia, both sympathetic and parasympathetic. A double-blind study showed that pyridostimine increases, on average, only 4 mm Hg in systolic BP.[87] The combination of 5 mg of midodrine with 60 mg pyridostigmine was slightly more effective than pyridostigmine alone. Similarly, the combination of pyridostigmine with atomoxetine appears to have a synergistic effect to increase blood pressure and improve orthostatic tolerance.[88]

Other agents such as the vasopressin analogue desmopressin (DDAVP), the centrally acting α2-antagonist yohimbine, the ergot alkaloid dihydroergotamine, and the nonselective adrenergic agonist pseudoephedrine are superseded and rarely used nowadays owing to their problematic adverse event profile.

NEUROGENIC SUPINE HYPERTENSION

The prevalence of neurogenic supine hypertension is 30% to 50% in Parkinson disease, 40% in MSA, and 50% to 70% in pure autonomic failure.[89] Treatment of supine hypertension focuses on reducing BP to lower the risk of target organ damage without worsening hypotension. Achieving this goal is challenging. Patients should avoid the supine position. For day naps, patients should sit in a reclining chair with the feet on the floor. At night, tilting the head of the bed to a 30° or a 45° angle lowers BP.[90] This is best accomplished with an electric bed or mattress. A carbohydrate-rich snack or an alcoholic drink before bedtime lowers BP. The application of a local abdominal heating pad to lower BP by inducing splanchnic vasodilation is being studied in a clinical trial (ClinicalTrials.gov: NCT02417415).

In patients with severe prolonged supine hypertension at night in spite of elevation of the head of the bed (systolic BP of at least 180 mm Hg or diastolic blood pressure of at least 110 mm Hg), short-acting antihypertensives (eg, captopril 25 mg, losartan 50 mg, or nitroglycerin patch 0.1 mg/h) at bedtime could be considered, particularly in patients who already have organ damage, although none of these approaches has been studied in large controlled trials.[24,91,92] Patients should be advised about the augmented risk of hypotension and falls if they stand up at nighttime (eg, to urinate). To avoid this, the use of a urinal or bedside commode should be encouraged.

SUMMARY

nOH is a disabling disorder that occurs frequently in patients with PD and other synucleinopathies. Mildly to moderately affected patients need a combination of nonpharmacological and pharmacologic therapies (eg, the synthetic mineralocorticoid fludrocortisone and the pressor agents midodrine or droxidopa). Severely affected patients are unable to stand but for a few seconds, making it impossible to perform even simple activities of daily living. The risk of falls and injuries is increased, and patients can become socially isolated because of the burden of symptoms. In these severe cases of nOH, success with available agents is only partial, and many patients continue to suffer severe symptoms. Exercise becomes intolerable, which inevitably leads to physical deconditioning and muscle atrophy, which, in turn, worsen the fall in BP. Despite its importance, there is a paucity of treatment options for this condition, the most recently available being droxidopa. New treatment options are needed.

REFERENCES

1. Woerman AL, Stohr J, Aoyagi A, et al. Propagation of prions causing synucleinopathies in cultured cells. Proc Natl Acad Sci U S A 2015;11:E4949–58.
2. Masuda-Suzukake M, Nonaka T, Hosokawa M, et al. Prion-like spreading of pathological alpha-synuclein in brain. Brain 2013;136:1128–38.
3. Prusiner SB, Woerman AL, Mordes DA, et al. Evidence for alpha-synuclein prions causing multiple system atrophy in humans with parkinsonism. Proc Natl Acad Sci U S A 2015;112:E5308–17.
4. Peelaerts W, Bousset L, Van der Perren A, et al. alpha-synuclein strains cause distinct synucleinopathies after local and systemic administration. Nature 2015; 522:340–4.
5. Peelaerts W, Baekelandt V. a-Synuclein strains and the variable pathologies of synucleinopathies. J Neurochem 2016;139(Suppl 1):256–74.
6. Marras C, McDermott MP, Rochon PA, et al. Survival in Parkinson disease: thirteen-year follow-up of the DATATOP cohort. Neurology 2005;64:87–93.
7. Halliday GM. Re-evaluating the glio-centric view of multiple system atrophy by highlighting the neuronal involvement. Brain 2015;138:2116–9.
8. Cykowski MD, Coon EA, Powell SZ, et al. Expanding the spectrum of neuronal pathology in multiple system atrophy. Brain 2015;138:2293–309.
9. Kaufmann H, Norcliffe-Kaufmann L, Palma JA, et al. Natural history of pure autonomic failure: a United States prospective cohort. Ann Neurol 2017;81:287–97.
10. Freeman R, Wieling W, Axelrod FB, et al. Consensus statement on the definition of orthostatic hypotension, neurally mediated syncope and the postural tachycardia syndrome. Clin Auton Res 2011;21:69–72.
11. Freeman R. Clinical practice. Neurogenic orthostatic hypotension. N Engl J Med 2008;358:615–24.
12. Masaki KH, Schatz IJ, Burchfiel CM, et al. Orthostatic hypotension predicts mortality in elderly men: the Honolulu Heart Program. Circulation 1998;98:2290–5.
13. Berganzo K, Diez-Arrola B, Tijero B, et al. Nocturnal hypertension and dysautonomia in patients with Parkinson's disease: are they related? J Neurol 2013; 260:1752–6.
14. Palma JA, Gomez-Esteban JC, Norcliffe-Kaufmann L, et al. Orthostatic hypotension in Parkinson disease: how much you fall or how low you go? Mov Disord 2015;30:639–45.
15. Velseboer DC, de Haan RJ, Wieling W, et al. Prevalence of orthostatic hypotension in Parkinson's disease: a systematic review and meta-analysis. Parkinsonism Relat Disord 2011;17:724–9.
16. Palma JA, Kaufmann H. Epidemiology, diagnosis, and management of neurogenic orthostatic hypotension. Mov Disord Clin Pract 2017;4:298–308.
17. Thaisetthawatkul P, Boeve BF, Benarroch EE, et al. Autonomic dysfunction in dementia with Lewy bodies. Neurology 2004;62:1804–9.
18. Kaufmann H, Goldstein DS. Autonomic dysfunction in Parkinson disease. Handb Clin Neurol 2013;117:259–78.
19. Jain S, Goldstein DS. Cardiovascular dysautonomia in Parkinson disease: from pathophysiology to pathogenesis. Neurobiol Dis 2012;46:572–80.

20. Goldstein DS, Holmes CS, Dendi R, et al. Orthostatic hypotension from sympathetic denervation in Parkinson's disease. Neurology 2002;58:1247–55.
21. Fuente Mora C, Palma JA, Kaufmann H, et al. Cerebral autoregulation and symptoms of orthostatic hypotension in familial dysautonomia. J Cereb Blood Flow Metab 2017;37(7):2414–22.
22. Horowitz DR, Kaufmann H. Autoregulatory cerebral vasodilation occurs during orthostatic hypotension in patients with primary autonomic failure. Clin Auton Res 2001;11:363–7.
23. Palma JA, Norcliffe-Kaufmann L, Kaufmann H. An orthostatic hypotension mimic: the inebriation-like syndrome in Parkinson disease. Mov Disord 2016;31:598–600.
24. Arnold AC, Biaggioni I. Management approaches to hypertension in autonomic failure. Curr Opin Nephrol Hypertens 2012;21:481–5.
25. Shibao C, Gamboa A, Diedrich A, et al. Acarbose, an alpha-glucosidase inhibitor, attenuates postprandial hypotension in autonomic failure. Hypertension 2007;50: 54–61.
26. Gibbons CH, Freeman R. Clinical implications of delayed orthostatic hypotension: a 10-year follow-up study. Neurology 2015;85:1362–7.
27. Cheshire WP Jr. Clinical classification of orthostatic hypotensions. Clin Auton Res 2017;27:133–5.
28. Bengtsson-Lindberg M, Larsson V, Minthon L, et al. Lack of orthostatic symptoms in dementia patients with orthostatic hypotension. Clin Auton Res 2015;25:87–94.
29. Norcliffe-Kaufmann L, Kaufmann H, Palma JA, et al. Orthostatic heart rate changes in patients with autonomic failure caused by neurodegenerative synucleinopathies. Ann Neurol 2018;83:522–31.
30. Norcliffe-Kaufmann L, Kaufmann H. Is ambulatory blood pressure monitoring useful in patients with chronic autonomic failure? Clin Auton Res 2014;24:189–92.
31. Umehara T, Matsuno H, Toyoda C, et al. Clinical characteristics of supine hypertension in de novo Parkinson disease. Clin Auton Res 2016;26:15–21.
32. Rose KM, Eigenbrodt ML, Biga RL, et al. Orthostatic hypotension predicts mortality in middle-aged adults: the Atherosclerosis Risk in Communities (ARIC) study. Circulation 2006;114:630–6.
33. Rose KM, Tyroler HA, Nardo CJ, et al. Orthostatic hypotension and the incidence of coronary heart disease: the Atherosclerosis Risk in Communities study. Am J Hypertens 2000;13:571–8.
34. Kamaruzzaman S, Watt H, Carson C, et al. The association between orthostatic hypotension and medication use in the British Women's Heart and Health Study. Age Ageing 2010;39:51–6.
35. Fotherby MD, Potter JF. Orthostatic hypotension and anti-hypertensive therapy in the elderly. Postgrad Med J 1994;70:878–81.
36. Biaggioni I, Robertson D, Krantz S, et al. The anemia of primary autonomic failure and its reversal with recombinant erythropoietin. Ann Intern Med 1994;121:181–6.
37. Perera R, Isola L, Kaufmann H. Effect of recombinant erythropoietin on anemia and orthostatic hypotension in primary autonomic failure. Clin Auton Res 1995; 5:211–3.
38. May M, Jordan J. The osmopressor response to water drinking. Am J Physiol Regul Integr Comp Physiol 2011;300:R40–6.
39. Low DA, Vichayanrat E, Iodice V, et al. Exercise hemodynamics in Parkinson's disease and autonomic dysfunction. Parkinsonism Relat Disord 2014;20:549–53.
40. Puvi-Rajasingham S, Smith GD, Akinola A, et al. Abnormal regional blood flow responses during and after exercise in human sympathetic denervation. J Physiol 1997;505(Pt 3):841–9.

41. Smith GD, Mathias CJ. Postural hypotension enhanced by exercise in patients with chronic autonomic failure. QJM 1995;88:251–6.
42. Smith GD, Watson LP, Mathias CJ. Neurohumoral, peptidergic and biochemical responses to supine exercise in two groups with primary autonomic failure: Shy-Drager syndrome/multiple system atrophy and pure autonomic failure. Clin Auton Res 1996;6:255–62.
43. Rowell LB. Human circulation: regulation during physical stress. New York: Oxford University Press; 1986.
44. Wieling W, van Lieshout JJ, van Leeuwen AM. Physical manoeuvres that reduce postural hypotension in autonomic failure. Clin Auton Res 1993;3:57–65.
45. Kooner JS, Raimbach S, Watson L, et al. Relationship between splanchnic vasodilation and postprandial hypotension in patients with primary autonomic failure. J Hypertens Suppl 1989;7:S40–1.
46. Jansen RW, Lipsitz LA. Postprandial hypotension: epidemiology, pathophysiology, and clinical management. Ann Intern Med 1995;122:286–95.
47. Pavelic A, Krbot Skoric M, Crnosija L, et al. Postprandial hypotension in neurological disorders: systematic review and meta-analysis. Clin Auton Res 2017;27: 263–71.
48. Goldstein DS, Cheshire WP Jr. Beat-to-beat blood pressure and heart rate responses to the Valsalva maneuver. Clin Auton Res 2017;27(6):361–7.
49. Krediet CT, van Lieshout JJ, Bogert LW, et al. Leg crossing improves orthostatic tolerance in healthy subjects: a placebo-controlled crossover study. Am J Physiol Heart Circ Physiol 2006;291:H1768–72.
50. Diedrich A, Biaggioni I. Segmental orthostatic fluid shifts. Clin Auton Res 2004;14: 146–7.
51. Smit AA, Wieling W, Fujimura J, et al. Use of lower abdominal compression to combat orthostatic hypotension in patients with autonomic dysfunction. Clin Auton Res 2004;14:167–75.
52. Fanciulli A, Goebel G, Metzler B, et al. Elastic abdominal binders attenuate orthostatic hypotension in Parkinson's disease. Mov Disord Clin Pract 2016;3:156–60.
53. Okamoto LE, Diedrich A, Baudenbacher FJ, et al. Efficacy of Servo-controlled splanchnic venous compression in the treatment of orthostatic hypotension: a randomized comparison with midodrine. Hypertension 2016;68:418–26.
54. Norcliffe-Kaufmann L, Axelrod FB, Kaufmann H. Developmental abnormalities, blood pressure variability and renal disease in Riley Day syndrome. J Hum Hypertens 2013;27:51–5.
55. Chobanian AV, Volicer L, Tifft CP, et al. Mineralocorticoid-induced hypertension in patients with orthostatic hypotension. N Engl J Med 1979;301:68–73.
56. Vagaonescu TD, Saadia D, Tuhrim S, et al. Hypertensive cardiovascular damage in patients with primary autonomic failure. Lancet 2000;355:725–6.
57. Grijalva CG, Biaggioni I, Griffin MR, et al. Fludrocortisone is associated with a higher risk of all-cause hospitalizations compared with midodrine in patients with orthostatic hypotension. J Am Heart Assoc 2017;6 [pii:e006848].
58. Jankovic J, Gilden JL, Hiner BC, et al. Neurogenic orthostatic hypotension: a double-blind, placebo-controlled study with midodrine. Am J Med 1993;95: 38–48.
59. Low PA, Gilden JL, Freeman R, et al. Efficacy of midodrine vs placebo in neurogenic orthostatic hypotension. A randomized, double-blind multicenter study. Midodrine Study Group. JAMA 1997;277:1046–51.
60. Wright RA, Kaufmann HC, Perera R, et al. A double-blind, dose-response study of midodrine in neurogenic orthostatic hypotension. Neurology 1998;51:120–4.

61. Smith W, Wan H, Much D, et al. Clinical benefit of midodrine hydrochloride in symptomatic orthostatic hypotension: a phase 4, double-blind, placebo-controlled, randomized, tilt-table study. Clin Auton Res 2016;26:269–77.

62. McTavish D, Goa KL, Midodrine. A review of its pharmacological properties and therapeutic use in orthostatic hypotension and secondary hypotensive disorders. Drugs 1989;38:757–77.

63. Kaufmann H, Norcliffe-Kaufmann L, Palma JA. Droxidopa in neurogenic orthostatic hypotension. Expert Rev Cardiovasc Ther 2015;13:875–91.

64. Kaufmann H, Biaggioni I. Autonomic failure in neurodegenerative disorders. Semin Neurol 2003;23:351–63.

65. Kaufmann H, Malamut R, Norcliffe-Kaufmann L, et al. The Orthostatic Hypotension Questionnaire (OHQ): validation of a novel symptom assessment scale. Clin Auton Res 2012;22:79–90.

66. Kaufmann H, Freeman R, Biaggioni I, et al. Droxidopa for neurogenic orthostatic hypotension: a randomized, placebo-controlled, phase 3 trial. Neurology 2014; 83:328–35.

67. Hauser RA, Isaacson S, Lisk JP, et al. Droxidopa for the short-term treatment of symptomatic neurogenic orthostatic hypotension in Parkinson's disease (nOH306B). Mov Disord 2015;30:646–54.

68. Elgebaly A, Abdelazeim B, Mattar O, et al. Meta-analysis of the safety and efficacy of droxidopa for neurogenic orthostatic hypotension. Clin Auton Res 2016;26:171–80.

69. Kaufmann H. Droxidopa for symptomatic neurogenic orthostatic hypotension: what can we learn? Clin Auton Res 2017;27:1–3.

70. Gupta F, Karabin B, Mehdirad A. Titrating droxidopa to maximize symptomatic benefit in a patient with Parkinson disease and neurogenic orthostatic hypotension. Clin Auton Res 2017;27:15–6.

71. Vernino S, Claassen D. Polypharmacy: droxidopa to treat neurogenic orthostatic hypotension in a patient with Parkinson disease and type 2 diabetes mellitus. Clin Auton Res 2017;27:33–4.

72. Kremens D, Lew M, Claassen D, et al. Adding droxidopa to fludrocortisone or midodrine in a patient with neurogenic orthostatic hypotension and Parkinson disease. Clin Auton Res 2017;27:29–31.

73. Mehdirad A, Karabin B, Gupta F. Managing neurogenic orthostatic hypotension with droxidopa in a patient with Parkinson disease, atrial fibrillation, and hypertension. Clin Auton Res 2017;27:25–7.

74. Claassen D, Lew M. Initiating droxidopa for neurogenic orthostatic hypotension in a patient with Parkinson disease. Clin Auton Res 2017;27:13–4.

75. Goodman BP, Claassen D, Mehdirad A. Adjusting droxidopa for neurogenic orthostatic hypotension in a patient with Parkinson disease. Clin Auton Res 2017;27:17–9.

76. Goodman BP, Gupta F. Defining successful treatment of neurogenic orthostatic hypotension with droxidopa in a patient with multiple system atrophy. Clin Auton Res 2017;27:21–3.

77. Gupta F, Kremens D, Vernino S, et al. Managing neurogenic orthostatic hypotension in a patient presenting with pure autonomic failure who later developed Parkinson disease. Clin Auton Res 2017;27:9–11.

78. Kaufmann H, Norcliffe-Kaufmann L, Hewitt LA, et al. Effects of the novel norepinephrine prodrug, droxidopa, on ambulatory blood pressure in patients with neurogenic orthostatic hypotension. J Am Soc Hypertens 2016;10:819–26.

79. Kaufmann H, Saadia D, Voustianiouk A, et al. Norepinephrine precursor therapy in neurogenic orthostatic hypotension. Circulation 2003;108:724–8.

80. Espay AJ, LeWitt PA, Kaufmann H. Norepinephrine deficiency in Parkinson's disease: the case for noradrenergic enhancement. Mov Disord 2014;29:1710–9.

81. Okamoto LE, Shibao C, Gamboa A, et al. Synergistic effect of norepinephrine transporter blockade and alpha-2 antagonism on blood pressure in autonomic failure. Hypertension 2012;59:650–6.

82. Shibao C, Raj SR, Gamboa A, et al. Norepinephrine transporter blockade with atomoxetine induces hypertension in patients with impaired autonomic function. Hypertension 2007;50:47–53.

83. Ramirez CE, Okamoto LE, Arnold AC, et al. Efficacy of atomoxetine versus midodrine for the treatment of orthostatic hypotension in autonomic failure. Hypertension 2014;64:1235–40.

84. Shibao C, Martinez J, Palma JA, et al. Norepinephrine levels predict the improvement in orthostatic symptoms after atomoxetine in patients with neurogenic orthostatic hypotension (P5.320). Neurology 2017;88.

85. Palma JA, Norcliffe-Kaufmann L, Martinez J, et al. Supine plasma NE predicts the pressor response to droxidopa in neurogenic orthostatic hypotension. Neurology 2018;91:e1539–44.

86. Jordan J, Shibao C, Biaggioni I. Multiple system atrophy: using clinical pharmacology to reveal pathophysiology. Clin Auton Res 2015;25:53–9.

87. Singer W, Sandroni P, Opfer-Gehrking TL, et al. Pyridostigmine treatment trial in neurogenic orthostatic hypotension. Arch Neurol 2006;63:513–8.

88. Okamoto LE, Shibao CA, Gamboa A, et al. Synergistic pressor effect of atomoxetine and pyridostigmine in patients with neurogenic orthostatic hypotension. Hypertension 2019;73:235–41.

89. Fanciulli A, Jordan J, Biaggioni I, et al. Consensus statement on the definition of neurogenic supine hypertension in cardiovascular autonomic failure by the American Autonomic Society (AAS) and the European Federation of Autonomic Societies (EFAS): endorsed by the European Academy of Neurology (EAN) and the European Society of Hypertension (ESH). Clin Auton Res 2018;28:355–62.

90. MacLean AR, Allen EV. Orthostatic hypotension and orthostatic tachycardia - treatment with the "head-up" bed. JAMA 1940;115:2162–7.

91. Kaufmann H, Palma JA. Neurogenic orthostatic hypotension: the very basics. Clin Auton Res 2017;27:39–43.

92. Di Stefano C, Maule S. Treatment of supine hypertension in autonomic failure: a case series. Clin Auton Res 2018;28:245–6.

Management of Urologic and Sexual Dysfunction in Parkinson Disease

Jason Margolesky, MD[a],*, Sagari Betté, MD[a,b], Carlos Singer, MD[a]

KEYWORDS

- Parkinson disease • Overactive bladder • Lower urinary tract symptoms
- Sexual dysfunction

KEY POINTS

- Urinary and sexual dysfunctions are common nonmotor symptoms in patients with Parkinson disease and they negatively affect the quality of life.
- Behavioral, medical, and procedural interventions are available for urinary and sexual dysfunction.
- Overactive bladder symptoms can be treated with anticholinergic agents or a beta-3 agonist (mirabegron), which has less potential adverse effects.
- Oral phosphodiesterase type 5 inhibitors and injectable prostaglandin E1analogues are available to treat erectile dysfunction.
- Management of urinary and sexual dysfunctions in women and men may differ, including treatment of diminished libido.

INTRODUCTION

Parkinson disease (PD) is defined by its motor manifestations: rigidity, tremor, bradykinesia, and postural instability. However, almost all patients with PD suffer from nonmotor symptoms that can be debilitating and may negatively affect quality of life more than motor symptoms.[1] Among the nonmotor manifestations, urinary and sexual dysfunctions are common[2] and potentially treatable.[3]

The PRIAMO study[4] included 1072 patients with PD (60% men; mean age 67 years). Nearly 60% complained of urinary symptoms, and the prevalence increased with disease severity from 43.1% prevalence in Hoehn and Yahr (HY) stage 1 to 89.8% in HY

Disclosures: Drs J. Margolesky and S. Betté have nothing to disclose. Dr C. Singer has received grants from Pharma2B, Sunovion, Adamas, Revance and honoraria from Abbvie and Mitsubishi.
[a] Department of Neurology, University of Miami Miller School of Medicine, 1150 Northwest 14th Street, Suite 609, Miami, FL 33136, USA; [b] Parkinson Disease and Movement Disorders Center of Boca Raton, 951 Northwest 13th Street, Suite 5E, Boca Raton, FL 33486, USA
* Corresponding author.
E-mail address: jhmargolesky@med.miami.edu

Clin Geriatr Med 36 (2020) 69–80
https://doi.org/10.1016/j.cger.2019.09.011
0749-0690/20/© 2019 Elsevier Inc. All rights reserved.

geriatric.theclinics.com

stage greater than or equal to 4. Urinary urgency, urinary frequency, and nocturia were present in 35%, 26%, and 34.6%, respectively. These lower urinary tract (LUT) symptoms are associated with increased fall risk[5] and lower Mini-Mental State Examination scores.[4]

In the same PRIAMO cohort, sexual dysfunction was present in 19.6%.[4] In men, erectile dysfunction (ED) and premature ejaculation were the most frequent problems.[6] Singer and colleagues[7] found that 60% of men with PD reported ED, compared with 37.5% of age-matched controls. Both men and women may endorse decreased libido.[6] Women with PD, when compared with aged-matched controls, are more likely to endorse vaginal tightness, loss of lubrication, involuntary urination, anxiety, and inhibition.[6] Increased libido has been reported as an adverse reaction to levodopa.[8] Compulsive sexual behavior can be a manifestation of impulse control disorder (ICD) induced by dopamine agonists; Weintraub and colleagues[9] reported that 3.5% of patients with PD using a dopamine agonist developed this side effect. Because patients are often not forthcoming regarding sexual symptoms, including hypersexuality as a manifestation of ICD and sexual dysfunction in general, practitioners are encouraged to ask all patients with PD about sexual dysfunction.

ANATOMY/PATHOPHYSIOLOGY
Neurology of Urinary Dysfunction

The LUT consists of the bladder, the urethra, and the intervening internal and external sphincters.[3] Normal function of the LUT involves the storage of urine and the voiding of urine at appropriate times. A center of micturition located in the pons controls the alternation of the storing phase (detrusor muscle relaxed, sphincters contracted) with the voiding phase (detrusor muscle contracted, sphincters relaxed—the micturition reflex).[10] Stimulation of receptors by sympathetic postganglionic noradrenergic neurons of the hypogastric nerve causes detrusor relaxation and sphincter contraction, resulting in bladder filling. Stimulation of receptors by parasympathetic postganglionic cholinergic neurons of the pelvic nerve causes detrusor contractions and bladder emptying.[3]

In PD, it has been theorized that the loss of basal ganglia output reduces cortical inhibition of the micturition reflex, leading to detrusor hyperactivity and excessive detrusor contractions, which underlie the symptom of urinary urgency.[11]

Neurology of Sexual Function

Penile erections are classified as reflex and psychogenic. Reflex erections occur in response to genital stimulation via sensory fibers of the dorsal penile nerve to the spinal cord (segments S2–S4).[10] From there, synaptic connections culminate in the parasympathetic cavernous nerves of the penis, releasing nitric oxide and triggering a chemical cascade that results in vasodilation of the penile arteries.[10] Psychogenic erections occur in response to visual, thought-based, and other erogenous stimuli that connect the conscious brain to the abovementioned sacral segments as well as, sequentially, to T11 to L2 segments, the splanchnic nerves, inferior hypogastric nerve, and the pelvic plexus.[10]

For ejaculation to occur, seminal vesicles and perineal muscles contract to propulse the ejaculate while simultaneously the urethral sphincters contract to prevent retrograde ejaculation into the bladder. Ejaculation is coordinated by sympathetic outflow from the spinal generator of ejaculation located in the L3 to L4 spinal segments.

In women, external genital stimulation is sensed through the dorsal clitoral nerve (afferent to the pudendal nerve) and transmitted to the sacral segments of the spinal cord, with eventual clitoral engorgement and vaginal lubrication.[10] This same pathway can be triggered by psychogenic inputs without physical stimulation.[10] For orgasm, women share with men a similar pathway.[10]

MANAGEMENT OF URINARY SYMPTOMS

The first step in managing urinary symptoms in PD is properly identifying the problem. This issue may be PD specific or related to problems common in the elderly, and formal urodynamic testing may be indicated to make an accurate diagnosis.

The common symptoms of benign prostatic hyperplasia (BPH)—bladder emptying difficulty (urinary retention and sensation of incomplete bladder emptying) or bladder storage difficulty (frequency, urgency, and nocturia)—can be expected in PD even without BPH.[12] However, bladder emptying difficulties in patients with PD without concomitant BPH are more likely related to other comorbid urologic or drug-induced causes or may even suggest the presence of a neurodegenerative disorder other than PD such as multiple system atrophy (beyond the scope of this review).[13–16]

Up to 45% of women older than 20 years have some degree of urinary incontinence, with daily episodes of incontinence affecting up to 40% of women older than 60 years.[17] The prevalence of urinary frequency, urgency, and incontinence in women increases around menopause (the same cohort as the general PD population) and aside from aging, may be related to hormonal changes[18] and anatomic changes of the pelvic floor musculature.[19] Female-specific treatment of urinary incontinence includes weight loss to take pressure off the pelvic floor, topical estrogens, and surgical treatments (bulking agents, slings, suspensions).[18,20] Kegel exercises and supervised pelvic floor therapy with biofeedback and electrostimulation have shown benefit in the treatment of stress and mixed urinary incontinence.[21,22]

Behavioral modifications can be instituted to improve symptoms of urgency: timed voiding, reduction of caffeine, alcohol and overall fluid intake, and voiding before bedtime.[14,20,23]

Medications to treat urinary urgency include antimuscarinic anticholinergics and an adrenergic beta 3 agonist (mirabegron). Mirabegron is preferred over antimuscarinics due to a better side-effect profile, particularly in patients with PD. In a retrospective study, 50 patients with PD received mirabegron, 50 mg, daily for 6 weeks and more than 60% reported improvement in nocturia and urinary urgency severity.[24] Only 2 adverse events (4%) were reported (1 patient with dizziness and 1 with diaphoresis).[24] In patients with PD and overactive bladder, 10 patients received solifenacin at a mean dose of 6 mg daily and 13 patients received placebo. The treatment group experienced a significant decrease in the number of urinary incontinence and nocturia episodes. Adverse events included constipation (11%), dry mouth (22%), and urinary retention (11%). No adverse events related to cognition were reported.[25] Solifenacin has greater selectivity to bladder muscarinic receptors (M3) compared with other anticholinergic agents,[25] which may account for the cognition-sparing side-effect profile. Furthermore, solifenacin may not negatively affect cognition in elderly patients with mild cognitive impairment.[26]

Anticholinergic side effects include xerostomia, constipation, dry eyes, blurred vision, and urinary retention.[27] However, most concerning in patients with PD (given their proneness to cognitive deficits) is an exacerbation of cognitive difficulty[28] and psychosis.[29–31] Although the pharmacologic properties of certain anticholinergic medications may mitigate this risk, this adverse event exists as a potential complication for any anticholinergics. Trospium, tolterodine, and darifenacin, as solifenacin, have low central nervous system (CNS) penetrance and are less likely to cause or aggravate cognitive dysfunction.[27,32] Oxybutynin and fesoterodine are less selective,[12] have moderate CNS penetrance, and are therefore less preferred.[27]

Posterior tibial nerve stimulation (PTNS) can improve detrusor overactivity and bladder capacity in patients refractory to or intolerant of oral medications for overactive bladder symptoms.[33,34] In a retrospective study, 33 patients with a neurologic disorder, including 4 with PD, were treated with PTNS.[35] Decreased nocturia was reported in 70% of that cohort. The therapeutic effect of the stimulation is presumed to come from neuromodulation and cross-signaling, as the posterior tibial nerve shares lumbosacral nerve roots with the nerves innervating the bladder.[33]

In cases of severe overactive bladder and urinary incontinence that have not responded to other treatments, onabotulinumtoxinA is approved by Food and Drug Administration (FDA).[12] All formulations of botulinum toxin prevent the release of acetylcholine by preventing synaptic vesicle docking, thereby preventing detrusor contractions. OnabotulinumtoxinA has been tested in patients with PD associated with urinary urgency secondary to detrusor muscle overactivity.[36–45] Doses ranged from 100 to 500 U injected into multiple sites within the detrusor muscle. The largest study included 20 patients with PD receiving 100 U and reported up to 6-month duration of effect in improving urinary symptoms.[39] Urinary retention is a possible adverse effect, in some cases requiring intermittent catheterization.[36–38]

Many medications can cause or contribute to urinary retention and should be discontinued. Medication classes to consider include anticholinergics, antiarrhythmics, antidepressants, antipsychotics, hormonal agents, muscle relaxants, and sympathomimetics.[46] Antiparkinsonian medications associated with urinary retention include amantadine, benztropine, and trihexyphenidyl.[46]

Chronic urinary retention and difficulty voiding in PD can be managed medically with α-1 blockers including alfuzosin, prazosin, doxazosin, tamsulosin, terazosin, and silodosin.[12] In a 12-week open-label study, 33 men with PD and voiding dysfunction received 4 mg per day of extended release doxazosin.[47] Doxazosin improved LUT symptoms, maximum flow rate, and quality of life in this cohort.[47] However, α-1 blockers can worsen postural hypotension, which is common in PD. Intermittent or chronic catheterization may be required, the latter via indwelling or suprapubic catheterization.

Patients with advanced PD may develop a functional type of incontinence based on immobility, fall risk, and dementia.[48] Treatments include keeping the path to the toilet lit and free of obstacles, bedside commodes and flasks, bed pads, and adult diapers.[14] Indwelling catheters pose infection risks but ultimately may be necessary. External "condom" catheters are available, which may be less cumbersome, the difference in infection risk is debatable, and the potential complication of penile strangulation and necrosis should be considered.

Table 1 summarizes the treatment options for urinary urgency, frequency, and nocturia. Mechanism of action, dosing instructions, and side effects are included.

MANAGEMENT OF DISORDERS OF SEXUAL PERFORMANCE
In Men

The contributions to successful sexual functioning include neurologic, vascular, endocrine, and psychosocial factors.[6,49] Sexual dysfunction is common in the general population; risk factors include age, smoking, diabetes, vascular disease, and other chronic diseases.[50,51] Compared with the general population, sexual dysfunction is more common in patients with PD, and, similarly to the general population, it is likely multifactorial.[2,49,52–59]

Table 1
Treatment options for overactive bladder symptoms including urinary urgency, frequency, and nocturia[27]

Medication	Mechanism of Action	Dosing Instructions	Side Effects
Mirabegron	Adrenergic beta 3 agonist	Start 25 mg once daily. After 8 wk can increase to 50 mg once daily Can be used concomitantly with solifenacin 5 mg once daily	Dizziness, diaphoresis, hypertension, irregular heart rate, abdominal or pelvic pain
Solifenacin	Anticholinergic	Start 5 mg once daily. Can increase to 10 mg once daily	Xerostomia, constipation, blurred vision, urinary retention, nausea, dyspepsia
Oxybutynin	Anticholinergic	Immediate release: 2.5 mg BID up to 5 mg QID Extended release: 5–15 mg once daily	Xerostomia, constipation, blurred vision, urinary retention, nausea, dyspepsia
Tolterodine	Anticholinergic	Immediate release: 2 mg BID Extended release: 2–4 mg once daily	Xerostomia, constipation, blurred vision, dyspepsia, dizziness, urinary retention
Fesoterodine	Anticholinergic	4–8 mg once daily	Xerostomia, constipation, blurred vision, dyspepsia, dizziness, urinary retention
Trospium	Anticholinergic	Immediate release: 20 mg BID Extended release: 60 mg once daily	Xerostomia, constipation, dry eyes, headache, urinary retention
Posterior tibial nerve stimulation (PTNS)	Neuromodulation	Unilateral stimulation	
Onabotulinum toxin A	Blocks presynaptic release of acetylcholine	100–200 units total every 12 wk	Urinary retention

In the case of both ED and ejaculatory dysfunction, PD medications should be optimized to maximize the motor requirements of sexual activity. However, many drugs, commonly used in the elderly, can negatively affect sexual function,[49] including, antidepressants (selective serotonin reuptake inhibitors [SSRIs]), thiazide diuretics, beta-adrenergic receptor blockers, and aldosterone antagonists, among others.[60,61]

Phosphodiesterase type 5 (PDE5) inhibitors via their action on nitric oxide vasodilation are established as an effective treatment of ED. In the case of PD, Raffaele and colleagues[62–65] reported improved erection in 84.8% of 33 patients receiving 50 mg of sildenafil daily. Other PDE5 inhibitors, such as tadalafil and vardenafil, also seem effective but lack formal studies in PD. These medications, however, should be avoided in patients with hypotension.[49] Intracavernous injections of alprostadil (prostaglandin E1) have proved effective in patients with neurogenic ED but have not been specifically tested in patients with PD. Injections are rapidly acting and may last from 2 to 4 hours. They require dexterity from the patient or partner, which may limit its utility in patients with PD.[49] For the medication averse, vacuum devices and constriction bands are available to address ED. These mechanical devices require dexterity that may limit their use in patients with PD. Finally, penile prostheses can be considered and require referral to urologic specialists.

For ejaculatory dysfunction, the drug regimen should be reviewed. Thiazide diuretics and alpha-blockers have been associated with retrograde ejaculation.[66] SSRIs are known to cause delayed ejaculation,[60] a side effect that may be helpful for patients with premature ejaculation.[49] Clomipramine has also been reported as useful for premature ejaculation.[49]

In Women

Women with PD have inadequate lubrication, may lose urine during sex, and may suffer anorgasmia.[49] Treatments include artificial lubricants, precoital voiding, and treatment of overactive bladder. In a study by Nurnberg and colleagues,[67] 49 women with depression, well-controlled with an SSRI but with subsequent sexual dysfunction, were randomized to placebo or sildenafil, 50 mg, (adjustable to 100 mg) before sexual activity. The treatment group had significant improvement in sexual function.

MANAGEMENT OF DISORDERS OF SEXUAL DESIRE (LIBIDO)

Testosterone deficiency in men with PD is of similar prevalence as in the general population (20%–25% of men aged 60 years or older) and can manifest with decreased libido and/or ED. Okun and colleagues[68] showed that a daily dose of transdermal testosterone gel improved symptoms in men with PD.

Flibanserin, a centrally acting serotonin agonist/antagonist is FDA approved for women with hypoactive sexual desire disorder (HSDD). In 3 randomized, double-blind, placebo-controlled trials, 1187 woman received flibanserin, 100 mg, at bedtime and 1188 patients received a placebo.[69–72] Flibanserin increased sexual desire, increased satisfying sexual events, and decreased distress associated with HSDD. Common side effects included dizziness, nausea, insomnia, somnolence, anxiety, and dry mouth. This and other pharmacologic measures have not been specifically studied in PD but can be considered.

Impulse control disorders (ICDs) affect up to 40% of patients with PD using dopamine agonists and about 15% of patients with PD overall.[73] ICDs include overeating, pathologic gambling, compulsive shopping, and hypersexuality. Compulsive sexual behavior can be defined as excessive and distressing sexual thoughts (or actions) persistent for more than 1 month and interfering with social activity.[74–76] The prevalence of compulsive sexual behavior is 4% in patients using dopamine agonists and about 2% in patients with PD not taking dopamine agonists.[74] Patients with PD should be screened for this behavior, so it can be promptly identified and managed. The mainstay of medical management for ICD is reducing or discontinuing dopamine agonists. Cognitive behavioral therapy was found to be "likely efficacious" and "possibly useful" for the treatment of ICD in patients with PD.[77]

Deep brain stimulation (DBS) is known to improve a number of nonmotor symptoms in patients with PD[78] but results for sexual dysfunction are mixed. Castelli and colleagues[73] reported improved satisfaction in sex life in men but not in women after subthalamic nucleus DBS. Some studies suggest improvement in ICDs after DBS, whereas others report de novo ICD occurring after surgery.[73]

Table 2
Treatment of sexual symptoms

Symptom	Medication	Mechanism of Action	Dosing Instructions	Side Effects
Erectile dysfunction	Sildenafil	PDE5 inhibitor	Start 50 mg once. May increase up to 100 mg up to once daily.	Hypotension, headache, flushing, dyspepsia, visual symptoms
	Tadalafil	PDE5 inhibitor	Start 10 mg once. May increase up to 20 mg up to once per 24 h. Alternative, for daily dosing: start 2.5 mg once daily. May increase to 5 mg once daily.	Hypotension, headache, flushing, dyspepsia, visual symptoms
	Vardenafil	PDE5 inhibitor	Start 10 mg once. May increase up to 20 mg up to once per 24 h.	Hypotension, headache, flushing, dyspepsia, visual symptoms
	Alprostadil	Prostaglandin E1	Start 1.25 mcg once. After 1 h may give 2.5 mcg once. After 24 h may give 5 mcg once. Maximum 2 doses per 24 h; maximum dose 60 mcg. May use more rapid titration for mixed causes (vascular/psychogenic/neurologic).	Priapism
	Mechanical devices	Mechanical/Structural	Varies based on device	Bruising, skin edema
Sexual dysfunction (women)	Sildenafil	PDE5 inhibitor	Start 50 mg once. May increase up to 100 mg up to once daily.	Hypotension, headache, flushing, dyspepsia, visual symptoms
	Flibanserin	Serotonin 5-HT1A agonist. Dopamine D4 and serotonin 5-HT2A, 5-HT2B, 5-HT2C antagonist.	Start 100 mg nightly. In premenopausal women, stop after 8 wk if no response.	Dizziness, nausea, insomnia, somnolence, anxiety, dry mouth
Sexual desire (men)	Testosterone	Androgen	30 mg every 12 h	Skin reactions, benign prostatic hypertrophy, testicular atrophy, hypertension, increased hematocrit, emotional lability

Table 2 summarizes the treatment options for sexual dysfunction. Mechanism of action, dosing instructions, and side effects are included.

SUMMARY

Urinary and sexual dysfunctions are common in PD as a result of PD itself, its treatment, and comorbid general medical conditions and their treatment. Treatment is optimal with a multidisciplinary approach, including pharmacologic and nonpharmacologic interventions, urologic and gynecologic specialists, and sex therapists. Treating urinary and sexual dysfunction can greatly improve the quality of life in patients with PD. Therefore, it is paramount that physicians inquire about these symptoms during routine visits so they can be elicited and addressed.

REFERENCES

1. Rahman S, Grifin HJ, Quinn NP, et al. Quality of life in Parkinson's disease: the relative importance of the symptoms. MovDisord 2008;23:1428–34.
2. Hand A, Gray WK, Chandler BJ, et al. Sexual and relationship dysfunction in people with Parkinson's disease. ParkinsonismRelatDisord 2010;16:172–6.
3. McDonald C, Winge K, Burn DJ. Lower urinary tract symptoms in Parkinson's disease: Prevalenc, aetiology and management. Parkinsonism RelatDisord 2017; 35:8–16.
4. Barone P, Antonini A, Colosimo C, et al. The Priamo study: a multicenter assessment of nonmotor symptoms and their impact on quality of life in Parkinson's disease. MovDisord 2009;24:1641–9.
5. Balash Y, Peretz C, Leibovich G, et al. Falls in outpatients with Parkinson's disease: frequency, impact and identifying factors. J Neurol 2005;252:1310–5.
6. Truong DD, Bhidayasiri R, Wolters E. Management of non-motor symptoms in advanced Parkinson disease. J NeurolSci 2008;266:216–28.
7. Singer C, Weiner WJ, Sanchez-Ramos IR, et al. Sexual function in patients with Parkinson's disease. J NeurolNeurosurgPsychiatry 1991;54:942.
8. Uitti RJ, Tanner CM, Rajut AH, et al. Hypersexuality in antiparkinsonian therapy. ClinNeuropharmacol 1989;12:375–83.
9. Weintraub D, Siderowf AD, Potenza MN, et al. Association of dopamine agonist use with impulse control disorders in Parkinson disease. Arch Neurol 2006;63: 969–73.
10. Daroff RB, Bradley WG. Bradley's neurology in clinical practice. Philadelphia: Elsevier/Saunder; 2012.
11. Zesiewicz TA, Evatt M, Vaughan CP, et al. Non-Motor Working Group of the Parkinson Study G, Randomized, controlled pilot trial of solifenacin succinate for overactive bladder in Parkinson's disease. Parkinsonism RelatDisord 2015;21: 514e520.
12. Sakakibara R, Panicker J, Finazzi-Agro E, et al. A guideline for the management of bladder dysfunction in Parkinson's disease and other gait disorders. NeurourolUrodyn 2016;35:551–63.
13. Simuni T, Sethi K. Nonmotor manifestations of Parkinson's disease. Ann Neurol 2008;64:S65–80.
14. Batla A, Phé V, De Min L, et al. Nocturia in Parkinson's disease: why does it occur and how to manage? MovDisordClinPract 2016;3(5):443–51.
15. Silva J, Silva CM, Cruz F. Current medical treatment of lower urinary tract symptoms/BPHL do we have a standard? CurrOpinUrol 2014;24:21–8.

16. Anderson BB, Pariser JJ, Helfand BT. Comparison of patient undergoing PVP versus TURP for LUTS/BPH. CurrUrol Rep 2015;16:55.
17. Buckley BS, Carmela M, Lapitan M. Prevalence of urinary incontinence in men, women, and children—current evidence: findings of the Fourth International consultation on incontinence. Urology 2010;76:265–70.
18. Hillard T. The postmenopausal bladder. MenopauseInt 2010;16:74–80.
19. Padmanabhan P, Dmochowski R. Urinary incontinence in women: a comprehensive review of the pathophysiology, diagnosis and treatment. Minerva Ginecol 2014;66:469–78.
20. Wood LN, Anger JT. Urinary incontinence in women. BMJ 2014;349:g4531.
21. Cavkaytar S, Kokanali MK, Topcu HO, et al. Effect of home-based Kegel exercises on quality of life in women with stress and mixed urinary incontinence. J ObstetGynaecol 2015;35:407–10.
22. Richmond CF, Martin DK, Yip SO, et al. Effect of supervised pelvic floor biofeedback and electrical stimulation in women with mixed and stress urinary incontinence. FemalePelvic Med ReconstrSurg 2016;22:324–7.
23. Hashimoto M, Imamura T, Tanimukai S, et al. Urinary incontinence: an unrecognized adverse effect with donepezil. Lancet 2000;356:*568*.
24. Peyronnet B, Vurture G, Palma J, et al. Mirabegron in patients with Parkinson disease and overacrive bladder symptoms: a retrospective cohort. Parkinsonism RelatDisord 2018;57:22–6.
25. Zesiewicz TA, Evatt M, Vaughan CP, et al. Randomized, controlled pilot trial of solifenacin succinate for overactive bladder in Parkinson's disease. Parkinsonism RelatDisord 2015;21:514–20.
26. Wagg A, Dale M, Tretter R, et al. Randomised, multicentre, placebo-controlled, double-blind crossover study investigating the effect of solifenacin and oxybutynin in elderly people with mild cognitive impairment: the SENIOR study. EurUrol 2013;64:74e81.
27. Palma J, Kaufmann H. Treatment of autonomic dysfunction in Parkinson disease and other synucleinopathies. MovementDisord 2018;33:372–90.
28. Ehrt U, Broich K, Larsen JP, et al. Use of drugs with anticholinergic effect and impact on cognition in Parkinson's disease: a cohort study. J NeurolNeurosurgPsychiatry 2010;81:160–5.
29. Hinkle JT, Perepezko K, Bakker CC, et al. Onset and remission of psychosis in Parkinson's disease: pharmacologic and motoric markers. MovDisordClinPract 2017;5(1):31–8.
30. Bennett N, O'Leary M, Patel AS, et al. Can higher doses of oxybutynin improve efficacy in neurogenic bladder. J Urol 2004;171:749–51.
31. Donnellan C, Fook L, McDonald P, et al. Oxybutynin and cognitive dysfunction. BMJ 1997;315:1363–4.
32. Jost WH. Urological problems in Parkinson's disease: clinical aspects. J NeuralTransm 2013;120(4):587e91.
33. de Wall LL, Heesakkers JP. Effectiveness of percutaneous tibial nerve stimulation in the treatment of overactive bladder syndrome. Res Rep Urol 2017;9:145–7.
34. Kabay SC, Kabay S, Yucel M, et al. Acute urodynamic effects of percutaneous posterior tibial nerve stimulation on neurogenic detrusor overactivity in patients with Parkinson's disease. NeurourolUrodyn 2009;28:62–7.
35. Wallace PA, Lane FL, Noblett KL. Sacral nerve neuromodulation in patients with underlying neurologic disease. Am J ObstetGynecol 2007;197:e1–5.

36. Giannantoni A, Rossi A, Mearini E, et al. Botulinum toxin A for overactive bladder and detrusor muscle overactivity in patients with Parkinson's disease and multiple system atrophy. J Urol 2009;182:1453–7.

37. Giannantoni A, Conte A, Proietti S, et al. Botulinum toxin type A in patients with Parkinson's disease and refractory overactive bladder. J Urol 2011;186:960–4.

38. Kulaksizoglu H, Parman Y. Use of botulinim toxin-A for the treatment of overactive bladder symptoms in patients with Parkinsons's disease. ParkinsonismRelatDisord 2010;16:531–4.

39. Anderson RU, Orenberg EK, Glowe P. OnabotulinumtoxinA office treatment for neurogenic bladder incontinence in Parkinson's disease. Urology 2014;83:22–7.

40. Rosa-Grilo M, Qamar MA, Taddei RN, et al. Rotigotine transdermal patch and sleep in Parkinson's disease: where are we now? NPJParkinsons Dis 2017;3:28.

41. Aranda B, Cramer P. Effects of apomorphine and L-dopa on the parkinsonian bladder. NeurourolUrodyn 1993;12:203–9.

42. Brusa L, Musco S, Bernardi G, et al. Rasagiline effect on bladder disturbances in early mild Parkinson's disease patients. ParkinsonismRelatDisord 2014;20:931–2.

43. Aranda R, Tateno F, Nagao T, et al. Bladder function of patients with Parkinson's disease. Int J Urol 2014;21:638–46.

44. Finazzi-Agro E, D'Amico A, Petta A, et al. Effects of subthalamic nucleus stimulation on urodynamic findings in patients with Parkinson's disease. J Urol 2003;169: 1388–91.

45. Seif C, Herzog J, van der Horst C. Effect of subthalamic deep brain stimulation on the function of the urinary bladder. Ann Neurol 2004;55:118–20.

46. Selius BA, Subedi R. Urinary retention in adults: diagnosis and initial management. Am FamPhysician 2008;77:643–50.

47. Gomes CM, Sammour ZM, de Bessa J, et al. Neurological status predicts response to alpha-blockers in men with voiding dysfunction and Parkinson's disease. Clinics (Sao Paulo) 2014;69:817–22.

48. Khandelwal C, Kistler C. Diagnosis of urinary incontinence. Am FamPhysician 2013;87:543–50.

49. Bronner G, Vodušek DB. Management of sexual dysfunction in Parkinson's disease. TherAdvNeurolDisord 2011;4(6):375–83.

50. Addis IB, Van Den Eeden SK, Wassel-Fyr CL, et al. Sexual activity and function in middle-aged and older women. ObstetGynecol 2006;107:755–64.

51. Laumann EO, Glasser DB, Neves RCS, et al. A Population-based survey of sexual activity, sexual problems and associated help-seeking behavior patterns in mature adults in the United States of America. Int J Impot Res 2009;21(3):171–8.

52. Celikel E, Ozel-Kizil ET, Akbostanci MC, et al. Assessment of sexual dysfunction in patients with Parkinson's disease: a case–control study. Eur J Neurol 2008;15: 1168–72.

53. Bronner G, Royter V, Korczyn AD, et al. Sexual dysfunction in Parkinson's disease. J Sex MaritalTher 2004;30:95–105.

54. Jacobs H, Vieregge A, Vieregge P. Sexuality in young patients with Parkinson's disease: a population based comparison with healthy controls. J NeurolNeurosurgPsychiatry 2000;69:550–2.

55. Zesiewicz TA, Helal M, Hauser MD. Sildenafil citrate (Viagra) for the treatment of erectile dysfunction in men with Parkinson's disease. MovDisord 2000;15:305–8.

56. Welch M, Hung L, Waters CH. Sexuality in women with Parkinson's disease. MovDisord 1997;12:923–7.

57. Wermuth L, Stenager E. Sexual problems in young patients with Parkinson's disease. ActaNeurolScand 1995;91:453–5.

58. Brown RG, Jahanshahi N, Quinn N, et al. Sexual function in patients with Parkinson's disease and their partners. J NeurolNeurosurgPsychiatry 1990;53:480–6.
59. Koller WC, Vetere-Overfield B, Williamson A, et al. Sexual dysfunction in Parkinson's disease. ClinNeuropharmacol 1990;13:461–3.
60. Waldinger MD, Hengeveld MW, Zwinderman AH, et al. Effecor of SSRI antidepressants on ejaculation: a double-blind, randomized, placebo-controlled study with fluoxetine, fluvoxamine, paroxetine, and sertraline. J ClinPsychopharmacol 1998;18:274–81.
61. Chrysant SG. Antihypertensive therapy causes erectile dysfunction. CurrOpinCardiol 2015;30:383–90.
62. Raffaele R, Vecchio I, Giammusso B, et al. Efficacy and safety of Fixed-dose oral sildenafil in the treatment of sexual dysfunction in depressed patients with Idiopathic Parkinson's disease. EurUrol 2002;41:382–6.
63. Hussain IF, Brady CM, Swinn MJ, et al. Treatment of erectile dysfunction with sildenafil citrate (Viagra) in parkinsonism due to Parkinson's disease or multiple system atrophy with observations on orthostatic hypotension. J NeurolNeurosurgPsychiatry 2001;71:371–4.
64. O'Sullivan JD, Hughes AJ. Apomorphine-induced penile erections in Parkinson's disease. MovDisord 1998;13:436–9.
65. Shulman LM, Taback RL, Rabenstein AA, et al. Non-recognition of depression and other non-motor symptoms in Parkinson's disease. ParkinsonismRelatDisord 2002;8:193–7.
66. Ralph DJ, Wylie KR. Ejaculatory disorders and sexual function. BJUInt 2005;95:1181–6.
67. Nurnberg HG, Hensley PL, Heiman JR, et al. Sildenafiltreatment of women with antidepressant-associated sexual dysfunction: a randomized controlled trial. JAMA 2008;300:395–404.
68. Okun MS, Walter BL, McDonald WM, et al. Benefical effects of testosterone replacement for the nonmotor symptoms of Parkinson disease. Arch Neurol 2002;59:1750–3.
69. DeRogatis LR, Komer L, Katz M, et al. VIOLET trial investigators. Treatment of hypoactive sexual desire disorder in premenopausal women: efficacy of flibanserin in the VIOLET study. J Sex Med 2012;9(4):1074–85.
70. Thorp J, Simon J, Dattani D, et al. DAISY trial investigators. Treatment of hypoactive sexual desire disorder in premenopausal women: efficacy of flibanserin in the DAISY study. J Sex Med 2012;9(3):793–804.
71. Katz M, DeRogatis LR, Ackerman R, et al. Efficacy of flibanserin in women with hypoactive sexual desire disorder: results from the BEGONIA trial. J Sex Med 2013;10(7):1807–15.
72. Stephen M. Stahl Mechanism of action of flibanserin, a multifunctional serotonin agonist and antagonist (MSAA), in hypoactive sexual desire disorder. CNSSpectr 2015. https://doi.org/10.1017/S1092852914000832.
73. Castelli L, Perozzo P, Genesia ML, et al. Sexual well being in parkinsonian patients after deep brain stimulation of the subthalamic nucleus. J NeurolNeurosurgPsychiatry 2004;75:1260–4.
74. Bhattacharjee S. Impulse control disorders in Parkinson's disease: review of pathophysiology, epidemiology, clinical features, management, and future challenges. NeuroIndia 2018;66:967–75.
75. Thomas A, Bonanni L, Gambi F, et al. Pathological gambling in Parkinson disease is reduced by amantadine. Ann Neurol 2010;68:400–4.

76. Walsh RA, Lang AE. Multiple impulse control disorders developing in Parkinson's disease after initiation of amantadine. MovDisord 2012;27:326.
77. Seppi K, Chaudhuri R, Coelho M, et al. Update on treatments for nonmotor symptoms of Parkinson's disease- an evidence-based medicine review. MovDisord 2019. https://doi.org/10.1002/mds.27602.
78. Kurtis MM, Rajah T, Delgado LF, et al. The effect of deep brain stimulation on the non-motor symptoms of Parkinson's disease: a critical review of the current evidence. NPJParkinsons Dis 2017;3:16024.

Gastrointestinal Care of the Parkinson Patient

John Legge, MD[a,b], Nicholas Fleming, MD[a,b], Leslie Jameleh Cloud, MD, MSc[b,c,*]

KEYWORDS

- Gastrointestinal symptoms • Constipation • Gastroparesis • Dysphagia • Drooling
- Weight loss • Parkinson disease

KEY POINTS

- Gastrointestinal symptoms such as weight loss, drooling, dysphagia, nausea, constipation, and defecatory dysfunction are common in patients with Parkinson disease.
- These symptoms negatively affect quality of life and can lead to serious or even life-threatening complications. Clinicians should therefore remain vigilant in identifying and treating them.
- Treatment should typically begin with a conservative nonpharmacological approach and escalate to pharmacotherapy as needed.
- The contribution of motor medication adverse effects should always be considered.

INTRODUCTION

Gastrointestinal (GI) symptoms are highly prevalent in Parkinson Disease (PD), reflecting dysregulation of motility at all levels of the GI tract. GI symptoms negatively impact quality of life[1–4] and may also lead to potentially life-threatening complications such as aspiration, malnutrition, megacolon, volvulus, intestinal obstruction, and possibly perforation.[5–10] Furthermore, they can affect other PD symptoms by interfering with levodopa absorption.[11–13] Clinicians should remain vigilant in screening for these GI symptoms so they can be managed aggressively. The clinical presentation, evaluation, and treatment

---

Disclosure Statement: Dr. Cloud had received a grant from the MJFF (Grant 11692). The other authors have nothing to disclose.
[a] Department of Neurology, Virginia Commonwealth University School of Medicine, Richmond, VA, USA; [b] VCU NOW Center, 11958 West Broad Street, 4th Floor, Box 980220, Henrico, VA 23298-0220, USA; [c] Parkinson's and Movement Disorders Center, Virginia Commonwealth University School of Medicine, Richmond, VA, USA
* Corresponding author. VCU NOW Center, 11958 West Broad Street, 4th Floor, Box 980220, Henrico, VA 23298-0220.
E-mail address: leslie.cloud@vcuhealth.org

Clin Geriatr Med 36 (2020) 81–92
https://doi.org/10.1016/j.cger.2019.09.003
geriatric.theclinics.com

options for the most common GI symptoms in Parkinson disease will be reviewed herein.

WEIGHT LOSS

Unintended weight loss is a frequently neglected nonmotor symptom that can negatively impact quality of life.[14,15] Longer disease duration, older age, and female sex have all been found to be associated with weight loss.[16–18] The etiology of weight loss in Parkinson disease is likely multifactorial including impaired olfaction and taste perception, dysphagia, gastroparesis, nausea and anorexia from dopaminergic drugs, and excessive caloric expenditure from hyperkinetic movements such as tremor and dyskinesia. A recent study found the extent of weight loss is correlated with the percentage of the waking day spent with dyskinesia.[19] As immobility worsens in later disease stages, loss of muscle mass (sarcopenia) also contributes to more dramatic weight loss.[20] Early detection of weight loss is critical to diminishing morbidity associated with malnutrition including infections, falls, fractures, and a decreased quality of life.[21]

Alternative medical causes should be ruled out in those experiencing dramatic weight loss, making consultation with primary care a critical first step. Concomitantly, referral to a registered dietician for evaluation of nutritional status and suggestions for dietary modification is often necessary to curtail weight loss.[21,22] If anorexia is a factor, understanding the root cause is important. Anorexia may reflect underlying gastroparesis, which may be levodopa-induced. Treatment of gastroparesis will be discussed. Occasionally, appetite stimulants may be needed. In patients with comorbid depression and/or insomnia, mirtazapine may be a convenient choice, although it has not been studied as an appetite stimulant in Parkinson disease. Other more traditional appetite stimulants such as megestrol or dronabinol can also be considered, although they have not been studied in Parkinson disease.

DROOLING

Drooling, defined as excessive pooling and poor control of saliva in the oral cavity, can have a profound effect on quality of life in Parkinson disease. The reported prevalence of drooling in patients with Parkinson disease varies considerably in the literature, ranging from 10% to 81%.[23] The negative sequelae of drooling include social embarrassment, poor oral hygiene and halitosis, difficulty eating and speaking, increased intraoral occult bacteria, and an increased risk of respiratory infection.[24,25] Interestingly, saliva production is not increased in Parkinson disease but is diminished,[26] which is why the authors prefer the term drooling over sialorrhea in the context of Parkinson disease. Drooling in Parkinson disease is thought to be the result of several mechanisms, including infrequent and inefficient swallowing, stooped posture, and the tendency for the mouth of Parkinson disease patients to remain open.[25,27] For the treatment of mild drooling, the use of chewing gum or hard candy in social situations can encourage swallowing and reduce pooling of saliva.[27] If more aggressive treatment is needed, the addition of topical and/or oral anticholinergics, adrenergic receptor agonists, or botulinum neurotoxin can be considered.

Sublingual ipratropium bromide spray (21 μg 4 times daily) improved subjective scores in a 2-week study but did not show objective differences when compared with placebo.[28] Alternatively, 1% atropine ophthalmic drops (1 drop sublingually twice daily) administered for 1 week demonstrated a statistically significant objective decline in salivary production with minimal risk of systemic adverse effects.[24,29] Although oral anticholinergic medications carry risks of adverse effects including cognitive dysfunction, urinary retention, and constipation, glycopyrrolate (1–2 mg twice to three times daily) has been shown to be effective and well-tolerated in short-term studies (<4 weeks) to reduce saliva production while minimizing adverse effects caused by its impaired ability to cross the blood-brain barrier.[30,31] Clonidine, an α-2 adrenergic receptor agonist, administered at 0.15 mg daily significantly reduced the number of times patients cleared their saliva when compared with placebo in a small, 3-month double-blind, placebo-controlled trial of 32 patients with Parkinson disease.[32] Botulinum toxin A or B injected into the parotid and submandibular glands is highly effective in diminishing salivary production, with effects lasting approximately 3 to 4 months.[24,33,34] **Table 1** summarizes pharmacologic treatment options for drooling in patients with Parkinson disease, including dosages and relevant adverse effect considerations.

DYSPHAGIA

Swallowing dysfunction is a frequent problem in patients with Parkinson disease and is an important risk factor for infection, malnutrition, hospitalization, and premature mortality. The prevalence of dysphagia in the Parkinson disease population has been reported to be up to 95% on objective testing and can be asymptomatic.[35] The use of modified barium swallow studies, videofluoroscopy, and esophageal manometry in Parkinson disease patients has identified multiple abnormalities in all 3 phases of swallowing (oral, pharyngeal, and esophageal), including delayed swallowing reflex, pyriform sinus residues, and aperistalsis.[22] These abnormalities can all lead to aspiration, which occurs in 15% to 56% of patients with Parkinson disease and underscores the importance of querying for aspiration symptoms during clinic visits.[27,36] Although prior small studies were unable to find a correlation between Parkinson disease severity and dysphagia, a recent study of 119 patients found that the severity of Parkinson disease as measured by the MDS-USPRS influences patients' ability to swallow medication.[37–39] Patients complaining of coughing or choking during meals should undergo further evaluation with a modified barium swallow (MBS) study in consultation with a speech and language pathologist. MBS cannot evaluate esophageal function; therefore, if the study is negative, further evaluation with videofluoroscopy is required.

Patients with confirmed aspiration risk should be treated by a speech and language pathologist for training on compensatory strategies such as expiratory muscle strength training, positioning and postural techniques, airway protection techniques, and adaptive dietary strategies if warranted.[40,41] Whether optimization of dopaminergic medications improves dysphagia remains controversial, but the authors believe it can sometimes be useful for oropharyngeal dysphagia.[42–44] Botulinum toxin or myotomy can be used effectively for cricopharyngeal dysfunction.[45] Rarely, gastrostomy feeding tube placement may be necessary for severe dysphagia with recurrent aspiration pneumonia.

GASTROPARESIS

Gastroparesis is a defined as the presence of appropriate symptoms for at least 12 weeks in association with delayed gastric emptying on scintigraphy and the absence of obstructive lesions on upper GI endoscopy. The true prevalence of gastroparesis in patients with Parkinson disease is unknown, because no studies have assessed it in an appropriately thorough and systematic way. Delayed gastric emptying (DGE), however, is a prominent nonmotor feature in all stages of Parkinson disease, with prevalence nearing 100%.[46] DGE causes a variety of nonspecific

Table 1
Recommended pharmacologic treatment of gastrointestinal problems in Parkinson disease

Symptom	Treatment	Dose	Adverse Effect Considerations	References
Drooling	Sublingual ipratropium bromide spray	1–2 sprays (containing 21 mcg per metered dose spray) as needed up to 4x/d	Dry nasal passages, epistaxis	Thomsen et al,[28] 2007
	Sublingual atropine ophthalmic 1% solution	1 drop 2x/d	Delirium, hallucinations	Hyson et al,[29] 2002
	Glycopyrrolate	1–2 mg 2-3x/d, maximum dose: 8 mg/d	Constipation, xerostomia, blurred vision, urinary retention, anhidrosis, palpitations, drowsiness, confusion	Arbouw et al,[31] 2010
	Clonidine	0.15 mg daily	Bradycardia, hypotension, drowsiness, headache	Chou et al,[32] 2007
	Abobotulinum toxin A	75–146.2 U per parotid gland, 78.7 U per submandibular gland	Xerostomia, dysphagia	Srivanitchapoom et al,[24] 2014
	Onabotulinum toxin A	5–50 U per parotid gland, 5 U per submandibular gland	Xerostomia, dysphagia	Ondo et al,[33] 2004
	Rimabotulinum toxin B	500–2000 U per parotid gland 250 U per submandibular gland	Xerostomia, dysphagia	Ondo et al,[33] 2004
Gastroparesis	Domperidone[a]	20 mg 4x/d	Elevated prolactin levels, sudden cardiac death	Soykan et al,[85] 1997
Constipation	Psyllium	5.1 g 2x/d	GI obstruction possible if not taken with adequate liquid	Ashraf et al,[72] 1997
	Polyethylene glycol	Up to 17 g daily	Electrolyte abnormalities may occur with chronic use	Zangaglia et al,[74] 2007
	Lubiprostone	Up to 24 mcg twice daily	Headache, hypotension, nausea, and vomiting	Ondo et al,[75] 2012
Defecatory dysfunction	Apomorphine	3–10 mg subcutaneous at first call to stool	Hypotension; pretreatment with an antiemetic is necessary	Mathers et al,[60] 1988; Edwards et al,[63] 1993
	Botulinum toxin A	100 U into puborectalis muscle using transrectal ultrasound guidance	Retreatment necessary	Albanese et al,[86] 1997

Only medications with published clinical trials in the PD population are listed.
[a] Not approved for use by FDA.

symptoms including nausea, vomiting, postprandial fullness, early satiety, and upper abdominal pain, and is frequently mistaken for other GI conditions.[47–49] Several studies have suggested that DGE contributes to motor fluctuations in patients who take levodopa, as levodopa must reach the small intestine for absorption.[11,12] Thus, motor fluctuations can also be a clue that the patient suffers from DGE. Parkinson disease patients with symptoms of DGE should undergo further diagnostic testing with either gastric emptying scintigraphy (GES), a gastric emptying breath test (GEBT), or a wireless motility capsule (WMC), all of which are now approved by the US Food and Drug Administration (FDA) for the diagnosis of gastroparesis. Consultation with a gastroenterologist to help diagnose and manage gastroparesis should be considered.

In those with suspected or confirmed gastroparesis, a gastroparetic diet should be adopted. This diet encourages small, frequent meals, avoidance of foods high in fat and fiber, taking fluids throughout meals, and remaining upright or walking for 1 to 2 hours after meals.[22] Unfortunately, pharmacologic therapies for gastroparesis in Parkinson disease are limited in the United States as the only FDA-approved medication, metoclopramide, is contraindicated in Parkinson disease, because it worsens parkinsonism through central dopamine blockade. Domperidone is a peripheral dopamine receptor blocker that does not cross the blood-brain barrier and therefore carries less risk of worsening parkinsonism. Although domperidone is available in many countries, it is not currently approved by the FDA. Although it has been used effectively in the Parkinson disease population for decades, domperidone is coming under increased scrutiny recently because of safety concerns, including concerns raised by a recent study finding a twofold increase in all-cause mortality in patients with Parkinson disease taking domperidone.[50,51] The authors strongly advise restricted use for refractory gastroparesis and then only with strict adherence to safety practices:

Dosing from 10 to 30 mg 4 times daily
Excluding patients with any clinically significant arrhythmia or prolonged QT interval
Safety monitoring every 2 months for the first year of use and every 6 months thereafter (to include physical examination, electrocardiogram [EKG], complete blood cell count [CBC], liver panel, renal panel, and concomitant medication review)
Providing the patient and all cotreating physicians with a list of medications that can interact with domperidone

Older, nonselective 5-HT4 receptor agonists such as cisapride have been shown to improve gastric emptying in Parkinson disease but have been withdrawn from the US market as a result of serious cardiac adverse effects caused by interactions with cardiac hERG channels, especially after metabolic inhibition of cytochrome P450 (CYP450) by comedications. They are now only available with restricted access in some countries.[23] Newer, highly selective 5-HT4 receptor agonists are currently in clinical development, including 1 ongoing trial in Parkinson disease.[52] Erythromycin, a motilin receptor agonist, is in widespread use (albeit off label) for gastroparesis but has not been studied rigorously in the Parkinson disease population. One small trial demonstrated a significant reduction in gastric emptying time as measured by WMC after a single dose of intravenous erythromycin.[53] Long-term use of erythromycin is limited by tachyphylaxis.[54] To mitigate the risk of tachyphylaxis, administration of oral erythromycin solution at a dose of 50 to 500 mg 3 times daily for 3 consecutive weeks, followed by 1 week off it, can be used in the gastroparesis population, including patients Parkinson disease. Erythromycin's use is further limited by drug-drug interactions with other drugs metabolized by CYP3A4.[22,55,56] Botulinum toxin injected into the pyloric sphincter can also be useful for refractory gastroparesis in some patients with an obstructive component to their gastroparesis, although it has not been studied in Parkinson disease specifically.[57] Gastric pacemaker placement may be beneficial for severe, refractory gastroparesis but has not been tested specifically in Parkinson disease.

DEFECATORY DYSFUNCTION

Defecatory dysfunction, defined as excessive straining, pain, or a feeling of incomplete evacuation, is present in up to two-thirds of patients with Parkinson disease and can present early in the disease course.[58,59] For effective defecation to occur, the action of several muscle groups must be coordinated. The internal and external anal sphincters and puborectalis muscles, those involved in fecal continence, must relax, while abdominal, diaphragmatic, and glottic muscles contract to increase intra-abdominal pressure. Multiple abnormalities in this complex process have been described, including paradoxic contraction of the sphincter muscles during defecation.[60,61]

Anorectal function can be formally evaluated using anorectal manometry, electromyography, and fluoroscopic defecography; however, these studies are neither routinely performed nor readily available at many medical centers. Despite its frequency, no specific treatments for defecatory dysfunction have been rigorously studied in the Parkinson disease population. Use of routine laxatives and stool softeners is generally not effective and may actually worsen symptoms.[62] Injection with the dopamine agonist apomorphine at first call to stool has been reported to improve defecation in patients with Parkinson disease; however, it has not undergone testing for long-term benefit, and the treatment can be difficult, requiring premedication with an antiemetic and possibly inducing orthostatic hypotension or other adverse dopaminergic effects.[63] Botulinum toxin injections into the external anal sphincter and/or puborectalis muscle have been reported to subjectively improve symptoms in over 50% of patients with Parkinson disease but must be repeated periodically under ultrasound guidance by a highly skilled practicioner.[64,65] Biofeedback training and pelvic floor physiotherapy have not been rigorously investigated in the Parkinson disease population but may be useful.[66] **Table 1** summarizes suggested pharmacologic treatment options for defecatory dysfunction in Parkinson disease, including dosages and relevant treatment considerations.

CONSTIPATION

Diminished bowel movement frequency, generally defined as fewer than 3 bowel movements per week, may occur in more than 50% of patients with Parkinson disease.[67] Stools may also be hard. The proposed mechanism is slowed transit through the colon, which can be up to twice as long in Parkinson disease versus controls, and may predate the motor features of the disease by several years.[68–70] The solid marker colon transit test and WMC are tests that can yield segmental colon transit times, but these are of limited utility in assessing constipation in Parkinson disease patients clinically.[71] Colonoscopy, if not up to date, may be needed to exclude other causes of constipation, particularly if any red flags are present in the history such as weight loss, rectal bleeding, fever, or anemia.

Management of constipation in PD should begin with conservative, nonpharmacological approaches such as increasing fluid intake, maximizing dietary fiber, and increasing daily activity levels. If possible, medications with the potential to exacerbate constipation should be stopped. If pharmacotherapy is required, psyllium, alone or in combination with a stool softener such as docusate sodium, is an effective and safe initial approach.[72] Should a more aggressive regimen be required, the addition of an osmotic laxative is preferred over other categories of laxatives because of their safety profile with long-term use. Polyethylene glycol is an osmotic laxative that has been specifically studied in patients with Parkinson disease and found to be effective.[73,74] Lubiprostone, an intestinal chloride secretagogue, enhances fluid secretion into the intestinal lumen, facilitating passage of softened stool through the gut. It was also found to be safe and effective for short-term treatment of constipation in Parkinson disease; however, because of its tendency to cause nausea as an adverse effect, it may not be well tolerated in individuals with comorbid gastroparesis.[75] Rectal laxatives such as biscodyl suppositories or sodium phosphate enemas can be utilized as rescue medications during severe periods of constipation.[76] **Table 1** summarizes suggested pharmacologic treatment options for constipation in patients with Parkinson disease, including dosages and relevant adverse effect considerations. Although no evidence exists to support their use in Parkinson disease, there are various newer prescription laxatives on the US market such as linaclotide, a guanylate cyclase-C agonist, and prucalopride, a 5-HT4 receptor agonist, which can be considered should the aforementioned approaches fail.

EFFECTS OF PARKINSON DISEASE THERAPIES ON GASTROINTESTINAL SYMPTOMS

Dopaminergic medications, the mainstay of medical treatment for Parkinson disease, can have both positive and negative effects on the GI tract. All dopaminergic medications can cause nausea and vomiting, which can limit their use. Dopaminergic medications also have a known inhibitory effect on upper GI motility, possibly worsening underlying gastroparesis, thereby contributing to GI symptoms such as nausea, vomiting, abdominal pain, early satiety, anorexia, and weight loss.[77,78] Conversely, dopaminergic medications may actually improve symptoms of sialorrhea, dysphagia, and anorectal dysfunction.[42,63,79] Excessive weight gain has been reported to occur, although rarely, as a result of compulsive eating in patients taking dopamine agonists.[80] Additional GI effects of medications commonly used in patients with Parkinson disease are listed in **Table 2**.

Deep brain stimulation (DBS) may also influence the expression of GI symptoms. Degluitition and constipation have both been reported to improve after subthalamic nucleus DBS.[81,82] Weight gain has also been observed after both bilateral and

Table 2
Gastrointestinal adverse effects of commonly used motor medications in Parkinson disease

Medications	Gastrointestinal Effects
Amantadine	Anorexia, constipation, diarrhea, dry mouth, dysphagia
Anticholinergics	Constipation, dry mouth, ileus, nausea, vomiting
Catechol O-methyltransferase inhibitors	Abdominal pain, anorexia, constipation, diarrhea, dry mouth, dyspepsia, flatulence, hepatic failure (tolcapone), nausea, vomiting
Dopamine agonists	Anorexia, abdominal cramps, constipation, diarrhea, dry mouth, dysphagia, epigastric pain, GI bleeding (bromocriptine), nausea, vomiting
Carbidopa/Levodopa	Abdominal pain, anorexia, constipation, diarrhea, dry mouth, dysphagia, nausea, vomiting, weight loss
Monoamine oxidase B inhibitors	Dry mouth, dyspepsia, nausea

unilateral subthalamic DBS surgery, and although further studies are needed, it has been suggested to result from suppression of chronic tremor and/or dyskinesia.[83,84]

SUMMARY

Vigilant screening by clinicians to identify and aggressively manage GI symptoms has the potential to greatly improve quality of life for patients with Parkinson disease. The contribution of Parkinson disease motor medications to the GI symptoms can be significant and should always be considered carefully. Although there are myriad treatments for some GI problems such as drooling and constipation, other problems such as gastroparesis and defecatory dysfunction have limited available treatment options. More research is needed to identify and test novel therapeutic approaches.

REFERENCES

1. Li H, Zhang M, Chen L, et al. Nonmotor symptoms are independently associated with impaired health-related quality of life in Chinese patients with Parkinson's disease. Mov Disord 2010;25(16):2740–6.
2. Visser M, Rooden S, Verbaan D, et al. A comprehensive model of health-related quality of life in Parkinson's disease. J Neurol 2008;255(10):1580–7.
3. Sakakibara R, Shinotoh H, Uchiyama T, et al. Questionnaire-based assessment of pelvic organ dysfunction in Parkinson's disease. Auton Neurosci 2001;92(1–2): 76–85.
4. Barone P, Antonini A, Colosimo C, et al. The PRIAMO study: a multicenter assessment of nonmotor symptoms and their impact on quality of life in Parkinson's disease. Mov Disord 2009;24(11):1641–9.
5. Robbins JA, Logemann JA, Kirshner HS. Swallowing and speech production in Parkinson's disease. Ann Neurol 1986;19(3):283–7.
6. Rosenthal MJ, Marshall CE. Sigmoid volvulus in association with parkinsonism: report of four cases. J Am Geriatr Soc 1987;35(7):683–4.
7. Caplan LH, Jacobson HG, Rubinstein BM, et al. Megacolon and volvulus in Parkinson's disease. Radiology 1965;85(1):73–9.
8. Kupsky W, Grimes M, Sweeting J, et al. Parkinson's disease and megacolon: concentric hyaline inclusions (Lewy bodies) in enteric ganglion cells. Neurology 1987;37(7):1253.
9. Bushmann M, Dobmeyer SM, Leeker L, et al. Swallowing abnormalities and their response to treatment in Parkinson's disease. Neurology 1989;39(10):1309.
10. Bird MR, Woodward MC, Gibson EM, et al. Asymptomatic swallowing disorders in elderly patients with Parkinson's disease: a description of findings on clinical examination and videofluoroscopy in sixteen patients. Age Ageing 1994;23(3): 251–4.
11. Kurlan R, Rothfield K, Woodward W, et al. Erratic gastric emptying of levodopa may cause "random" fluctuations of parkinsonian mobility. Neurology 1988; 38(3):419.
12. Djaldetti R, Baron J, Ziv I, et al. Gastric emptying in Parkinson's disease: patients with and without response fluctuations. Neurology 1996;46(4):1051–4.
13. Djaldetti R, Achiron A, Ziv I, et al. First emergence of "delayed-on" and "dose failure" phenomena in a patient with Parkinson's disease following vagotomy. Mov Disord 1994;9(5):582–3.
14. Akbar U, He Y, Dai Y, et al. Weight loss and impact on quality of life in Parkinson's disease. PLoS One 2015;10(5).

15. Wills A-MA, Pérez A, Wang J, et al. Association between change in body mass index, unified Parkinson's disease rating scale scores, and survival among persons with parkinson disease: secondary analysis of longitudinal data from NINDS exploratory trials in Parkinson disease long-term study 1. JAMA Neurol 2016; 73(3):321.

16. Cersosimo MG, Raina GB, Pellene LA, et al. Weight loss in Parkinson's disease: the relationship with motor symptoms and disease progression. Biomed Res Int 2018;2018:9642524.

17. Durrieu G, Llau M-E, Rascol O, et al. Parkinson's disease and weight loss: a study with anthropometric and nutritional assessment. Clin Auton Res 1992;2(3):153–7.

18. Jaafar AF, Gray WK, Porter B, et al. A cross-sectional study of the nutritional status of community-dwelling people with idiopathic Parkinson's disease. BMC Neurol 2010;10:124.

19. Fabbri M, Zibetti M, Beccaria L, et al. Levodopa/carbidopa intestinal gel infusion and weight loss in Parkinson's disease. Eur J Neurol 2019;26(3):490–6.

20. Vetrano DL, Pisciotta MS, Laudisio A, et al. Sarcopenia in Parkinson disease: comparison of different criteria and association with disease severity. J Am Med Dir Assoc 2018;19(6):523–7.

21. Ma K, Xiong N, Shen Y, et al. Weight loss and malnutrition in patients with Parkinson's disease: current knowledge and future prospects. Front Aging Neurosci 2018;10:1.

22. Cloud L, Greene J. Gastrointestinal features of Parkinson's disease. Curr Neurol Neurosci Rep 2011;11(4):379–84.

23. Fasano A, Visanji NP, Liu LWC, et al. Gastrointestinal dysfunction in Parkinson's disease. Lancet Neurol 2015;14(6):625–39.

24. Srivanitchapoom P, Pandey S, Hallett M. Drooling in Parkinson's disease: a review. Parkinsonism Relat Disord 2014;20(11):1109–18.

25. Nóbrega AC, Rodrigues B, Melo A. Is silent aspiration a risk factor for respiratory infection in Parkinson's disease patients? Parkinsonism Relat Disord 2008;14(8): 646–8.

26. Tumilasci OR, Cersósimo MG, Belforte JE, et al. Quantitative study of salivary secretion in Parkinson's disease. Mov Disord 2006;21(5):660–7.

27. Pfeiffer RF. Gastrointestinal dysfunction in Parkinson's disease. Parkinsonism Relat Disord 2011;17(1):10–5.

28. Thomsen TR, Galpern WR, Asante A, et al. Ipratropium bromide spray as treatment for sialorrhea in Parkinson's disease. Mov Disord 2007;22(15):2268–73.

29. Hyson HC, Johnson AM, Jog MS. Sublingual Atropine for sialorrhea secondary to parkinsonism: a pilot study. Mov Disord 2002;17(6):1318–20.

30. Seppi K, Weintraub D, Coelho M, et al. The movement disorder Society evidence-based medicine review update: treatments for the non-motor symptoms of Parkinson's disease. Mov Disord 2011;26(S3):S42–80.

31. Arbouw MEL, Movig KLL, Koopmann M, et al. Glycopyrrolate for sialorrhea in Parkinson disease: a randomized, double-blind, crossover trial. Neurology 2010; 74(15):1203–7.

32. Chou KL, Evatt M, Hinson V, et al. Sialorrhea in Parkinson's disease: a review. Mov Disord 2007;22(16):2306–13.

33. Ondo GW, Hunter GC, Moore GW. A double-blind placebo-controlled trial of botulinum toxin B for sialorrhea in Parkinson's disease. Neurology 2004;62(1):37–40.

34. Lagalla G, Millevolte M, Capecci M, et al. Botulinum toxin type A for drooling in Parkinson's disease: a double-blind, randomized, placebo-controlled study. Mov Disord 2006;21(5):704–7.

35. Nienstedt JC, Bihler M, Niessen A, et al. Predictive clinical factors for penetration and aspiration in Parkinson's disease. Neurogastroenterol Motil 2018;31(3): e13524.

36. Lin C-W, Chang Y-C, Chen W-S, et al. Prolonged swallowing time in dysphagic parkinsonism patients with aspiration pneumonia. Arch Phys Med Rehabil 2012;93(11):2080–4.

37. Buhmann C, Bihler M, Emich K, et al. Pill swallowing in Parkinson's disease: a prospective study based on flexible endoscopic evaluation of swallowing. Parkinsonism Relat Disord 2019;62:51–6.

38. Ali G, Wallace K, Schwartz R, et al. Mechanisms of oral-pharyngeal dysphagia in patients with Parkinson's disease. Gastroenterology 1996;110(2):383–92.

39. Castell JA, Johnston BT, Colcher A, et al. Manometric abnormalities of the oesophagus in patients with Parkinson's disease. Neurogastroenterol Motil 2001;13(4):361–4.

40. Suttrup I, Warnecke T. Dysphagia in Parkinson's disease. Dysphagia 2016;31(1): 24–32.

41. Troche MS, Okun MS, Rosenbek JC, et al. Aspiration and swallowing in Parkinson disease and rehabilitation with EMST: a randomized trial. Neurology 2010;75(21): 1912–9.

42. Fuh J-L, Lee R-C, Wang S-J, et al. Swallowing difficulty in Parkinson's disease. Clin Neurol Neurosurg 1997;99(2):106–12.

43. Menezes C, Melo A. Does levodopa improve swallowing dysfunction in Parkinson's disease patients? J Clin Pharm Ther 2009;34(6):673–6.

44. Warnecke T, Suttrup I, Schröder JB, et al. Levodopa responsiveness of dysphagia in advanced Parkinson's disease and reliability testing of the FEES-Levodopa-test. Parkinsonism Relat Disord 2016;28:100–6.

45. Pfeiffer R. Management of autonomic dysfunction in Parkinson's disease. Semin Neurol 2017;37(2):176–85.

46. Goetze O, Nikodem AB, Wiezcorek J, et al. Predictors of gastric emptying in Parkinson's disease. Neurogastroenterol Motil 2006;18(5):369–75.

47. Soykan I, Sivri B, Sarosiek I, et al. Demography, clinical characteristics, psychological and abuse profiles, treatment, and long-term follow-up of patients with gastroparesis. Dig Dis Sci 1998;43(11):2398–404.

48. Hoogerwerf WA, Pasricha PJ, Kalloo AN, et al. Pain: the overlooked symptom in gastroparesis. Am J Gastroenterol 1999;94(4):1029.

49. Anaparthy R, Pehlivanov N, Grady J, et al. Gastroparesis and gastroparesis-like syndrome: response to therapy and its predictors. Dig Dis Sci 2009;54(5): 1003–10.

50. Simeonova M, Vries F, Pouwels S, et al. Increased risk of all-cause mortality associated with domperidone use in Parkinson's patients: a population-based cohort study in the UK. Br J Clin Pharmacol 2018;84(11):2551–61.

51. Rossi M, Giorgi G. Domperidone and long QT syndrome. Curr Drug Saf 2010; 5(3):257–62.

52. Cloud L, Norris V, Blackwell G, et al. RQ-00000010 for gastroparesis in Parkinson's disease: a single ascending dose study. Poster presented at: Parkinson Study Group 2019. Mov Disord 2019;34(S1):S16.

53. Rinonos S, Hoder J, Norris V, et al. Prokinetic pharmacologic intervention as a novel method for optimization of levodopa pharmacokinetics and pharmacodynamics in Parkinson's disease: results from a pilot study using erythromycin. Poster presented at: world Parkinson congress 2016. J Parkinsons Dis 2016;6(Suppl 1):1–284.

54. Richards RD, Davenport K, McCallum RW. The treatment of idiopathic and diabetic gastroparesis with acute intravenous and chronic oral erythromycin. Am J Gastroenterol 1993;88(2):203–7.
55. Acosta A, Camilleri M. Prokinetics in gastroparesis. Gastroenterol Clin North Am 2015;44(1):97–111.
56. Ray WA, Murray KT, Meredith S, et al. Oral erythromycin and the risk of sudden death from cardiac causes. N Engl J Med 2004;351(11):1089–96.
57. Ukleja A, Tandon K, Shah K, et al. Endoscopic botox injections in therapy of refractory gastroparesis. World J Gastrointest Endosc 2015;7(8):790–8.
58. Edwards LL, Pfeiffer RF, Quigley EMM, et al. Gastrointestinal symptoms in Parkinson's disease. Mov Disord 1991;6(2):151–6.
59. Bassotti G, Maggio D, Battaglia E, et al. Manometric investigation of anorectal function in early and late stage Parkinson's disease. J Neurol Neurosurg Psychiatry 2000;68(6):768.
60. Mathers SE, Kempster PA, Swash M, et al. Constipation and paradoxical puborectalis contraction in anismus and Parkinson's disease: a dystonic phenomenon? J Neurol Neurosurg Psychiatry 1988;51(12):1503.
61. Mathers S, Kempster PA, Law P, et al. Anal sphincter dysfunction in Parkinson's disease. Arch Neurol 1989;46(10):1061–4.
62. Pfeiffer RF. Gastrointestinal dysfunction in Parkinson's disease. Lancet Neurol 2003;2(2):107–16.
63. Edwards LL, Quigley EMM, Harned RK, et al. Defecatory function in Parkinson's disease: response to apomorphine. Ann Neurol 1993;33(5):490–3.
64. Albanese RA, Brisinda RG, Bentivoglio RA, et al. Treatment of outlet obstruction constipation in Parkinson's disease with botulinum neurotoxin A. Am J Gastroenterol 2003;98(6):1439–40.
65. Cadeddu F, Bentivoglio AR, Brandara F, et al. Outlet type constipation in Parkinson's disease: results of botulinum toxin treatment. Aliment Pharmacol Ther 2005; 22(10):997–1003.
66. Rao SSC. Dyssynergic defecation and biofeedback therapy. Gastroenterol Clin North Am 2008;37(3):569–86.
67. Edwards L, Quigley EMM, Hofman R, et al. Gastrointestinal symptoms in Parkinson disease: 18-month follow-up study. Mov Disord 1993;8(1):83–6.
68. Edwards LL, Quigley EM, Harned RK, et al. Characterization of swallowing and defecation in Parkinson's disease. Am J Gastroenterol 1994;89(1).
69. Jost W, Schrank B. Defecatory disorders in de novo Parkinsonians–colonic transit and electromyogram of the external anal sphincter. Wien Klin Wochenschr 1998; 110(15):535–7.
70. Sakakibara R, Odaka T, Uchiyama T, et al. Colonic transit time, sphincter EMG, and rectoanal videomanometry in multiple system atrophy. Mov Disord 2004; 19(8):924–9.
71. Lin H, Prather C, Fisher R, et al. Measurement of gastrointestinal transit. Dig Dis Sci 2005;50(6):989–1004.
72. Ashraf W, Pfeiffer RF, Park F, et al. Constipation in Parkinson's disease: objective assessment and response to psyllium. Mov Disord 1997;12(6):946–51.
73. Eichhorn TE, Oertel WH. Macrogol 3350/electrolyte improves constipation in Parkinson's disease and multiple system atrophy. Mov Disord 2001;16(6):1176–7.
74. Zangaglia R, Martignoni E, Glorioso M, et al. Macrogol for the treatment of constipation in Parkinson's disease. A randomized placebo-controlled study. Mov Disord 2007;22(9):1239–44.

75. Ondo WG, Kenney C, Sullivan K, et al. Placebo-controlled trial of lubiprostone for constipation associated with Parkinson disease. Neurology 2012;78(21):1650–4.
76. Rossi M, Merello M, Perez-Lloret S. Management of constipation in Parkinsons disease, vol. 16. London: Informa UK, Ltd; 2015. p. 547–57.
77. Wiley J, Owyang C. Dopaminergic modulation of rectosigmoid motility: action of domperidone. J Pharmacol Exp Ther 1987;242(2):548.
78. Hardoff R, Sula M, Tamir A, et al. Gastric emptying time and gastric motility in patients with Parkinson's disease. Mov Disord 2001;16(6):1041.
79. Tison F, Wiart L, Guatterie M, et al. Effects of central dopaminergic stimulation by apomorphine on swallowing disorders in Parkinson's disease. Mov Disord 1996; 11(6):729–32.
80. Nirenberg MJ, Waters C. Compulsive eating and weight gain related to dopamine agonist use. Mov Disord 2006;21(4):524–9.
81. Ciucci MR, Barkmeier-Kraemer JM, Sherman SJ. Subthalamic nucleus deep brain stimulation improves deglutition in Parkinson's disease. Mov Disord 2008; 23(5):676–83.
82. Zibetti M, Torre E, Cinquepalmi A, et al. Motor and nonmotor symptom follow-up in parkinsonian patients after deep brain stimulation of the subthalamic nucleus. Eur Neurol 2007;58(4):218–23.
83. Tuite PJ, Maxwell RE, Ikramuddin S, et al. Weight and body mass index in Parkinson's disease patients after deep brain stimulation surgery. Parkinsonism Relat Disord 2005;11(4):247–52.
84. Walker HC, Lyerly M, Lee E, et al. Weight changes associated with unilateral STN DBS and advanced PD. Neurology 2009;72(11):A223.
85. Soykan I, Sarosiek I, Shifflett J, et al. Effect of chronic oral domperidone therapy on gastrointestinal symptoms and gastric emptying in patients with Parkinson's disease. Mov Disord 1997;12(6):952–7.
86. Albanese A, Maria G, Bentivoglio AR, et al. Severe constipation in Parkinson's disease relieved by botulinum toxin. Mov Disord 1997;12(5):764–6.

Depression and Anxiety in Parkinson Disease

Sudeshna Ray, MD[a], Pinky Agarwal, MD[a,b],*

KEYWORDS

- Depression • Anxiety • Parkinson disease • Quality of life
- Neuropsychiatric complication

KEY POINTS

- Depression and anxiety are the most common neuropsychiatric complications in Parkinson disease, which negatively impacts quality of life and increases caregiver burden.
- The symptoms of depression and anxiety overlap with that of Parkinson disease and may go unrecognized.
- Anxiety delays therapeutic response to antidepressants.
- In Parkinson disease, depression and anxiety often coexist.
- Multidisciplinary intervention strategies optimize patient response.

INTRODUCTION

Depression and anxiety are common psychiatric comorbidities in Parkinson disease (PD), which contribute to significant functional impairment[1] and adversely affect motor and social performance. This leads to poor quality of life[2–6] and increased caregiver burden.

Mood disorders are often under-recognized because symptoms overlap with cognitive and motor features of PD.[7,8] Therefore, early detection and optimal therapy for anxiety and depression is important in the management of PD.

EPIDEMIOLOGY

Depressive symptoms in PD are reported in approximately 20% to 30% of patients.[9] Depression may present before the clinical diagnosis of PD is made.[10] Clinically significant anxiety symptoms occur in 20% to 52% of patients.[11–14] Anxiety may be a

Disclosure Statement: Dr P. Agarwal received funding from Adamas, Ammneal and US World-Meds. Dr S. Ray has nothing to disclose.
[a] Booth Gardner Parkinson's Care Center, Evergreen Neuroscience Institute, 12039 NE 128th St, MS-77, Kirkland, WA 98034, USA; [b] University of Washington, Seattle, WA, USA
* Corresponding author. Clinical Professor, University of Washington, Booth Gardner Parkinson's Center, Evergreen Neuroscience Institute, 12039 NE 128th St, MS-77, Kirkland, WA 98034, USA.
E-mail address: pagarwal@evergreenhealth.com

Clin Geriatr Med 36 (2020) 93–104
https://doi.org/10.1016/j.cger.2019.09.012
0749-0690/20/© 2019 Elsevier Inc. All rights reserved.

result of the neurochemical changes of the disease itself or a psychological reaction to the stress of the disease.[14] In most patients, anxiety and depression coexist.[15]

In the PROMS-PD study, depression was strongly related to axial motor symptoms, whereas anxiety was commonly seen in younger patients ($\leq$55 years) and in those with motor fluctuations.[16,17]

CLASSIFICATION

The diagnosis of depression and anxiety disorders in PD is based on the *Diagnostic and Statistical Manual of Mental Disorders* V criteria by the American Psychiatric Association.

Types of depressive disorders seen in PD include[18]:

- Major depression: Persistence and general pervasiveness of 5 of 9 potential symptoms of which at least one of the symptoms should be either (1) depressed mood or (2) loss of interest or pleasure during the same 2-week period that represent a change from previous functioning. The symptoms are present most of the day, nearly every day.
  - Depressed mood
  - Markedly diminished interest or pleasure in all, or almost all, activities
  - Loss or gain in weight or appetite
  - Insomnia or hypersomnia
  - Psychomotor agitation or retardation
  - Fatigue or loss of energy
  - Feelings of worthlessness or excessive or inappropriate guilt
  - Diminished ability to think or concentrate, or indecisiveness
  - Recurrent thoughts of death, recurrent suicidal ideation without a specific plan, or a suicide attempt or a specific plan for committing suicide.
- Minor depression: Two of the 9 symptoms mentioned for major depression, but one must be either depression/sadness or loss of interest/pleasure. Patients with minor depressive disorder suffer from significant depressive symptoms interfering in their lives.
- Dysthymia: Dysthymia, now called persistent depressive disorder in the *Diagnostic and Statistical Manual of Mental Disorders* V, represents major depressive disorder lasting for at least 2 years.
- Subsyndromal depression: There are no uniformly accepted criteria for subsyndromal depression. It involves the presence of 2 or more depressive symptoms at a subthreshold level. Subthreshold level mean that symptoms are of "short duration" or are not "present most of the day" or "nearly every day."[7]

Anxiety may present as panic attacks, phobias, or generalized anxiety disorder. Anxiety and depression in PD may be episodic, often worsening during off periods, or continuous.

RISK FACTORS FOR DEPRESSION AND ANXIETY

Risk factors for depression
- Genetic: Depression is more common among patients with PD who are carriers of the Gly2019Ser mutation in the LRRK2 gene, when compared with no carriers.[19] A longitudinally followed PD population with GBA mutation was found to have increased scores of depression.[20]
- Women
- Advanced stages of PD

- Cognitive impairment[21]

Risk factors for anxiety

- Depressive symptoms
- Insomnia
- Dysautonomia
- Cognitive impairment
- Truncal imbalance and gait disturbances
- Motor fluctuations and off time[22]

SCALES
Depression Assessment Scales

The American Academy of Neurology in 2006 concluded that the Beck Depression Inventory, Hamilton Depression Rating Scale, and Montgomery–Asberg Depression Rating Scale had the highest diagnostic accuracy and were sufficient to screen patients with PD (evidence level B).[23]

For the purpose of screening depression in PD, a 2007 MDS Task Force review concluded that the Hamilton Depression Rating Scale, Beck Depression Inventory, Hospital Anxiety and Depression Scale, Montgomery–Asberg Depression Rating, and Geriatric depression scale are appropriate as screening scales for depression in PD.[24]

Anxiety Assessment Scales

The 3 most commonly applied anxiety assessment scales validated for use in PD are the Beck Anxiety Inventory, the Hospital Anxiety and Depression Scale, and the Hamilton Anxiety Rating Scale.[25]

PHARMACOLOGIC INTERVENTION
Depression

Treatment strategies range from counseling to pharmacologic intervention.[26] A few commonly used antidepressants in PD are discussed in **Table 1**. The SAD PD trial provided class 1 evidence that paroxetine and venlafaxine XR are effective in treating depression in patients with PD.[27]

Treatment Strategy

- Screen for underlying metabolic disturbances, which can mimic depression. A serum vitamin B_{12} level, thyroid function tests, and complete blood count may be performed. Screening for hypogonadism is recommended in males with refractory depression.
- Psychosocial issues may be referred for counseling.
- Balanced nutrition with adequate caloric intake should be encouraged.
- Regular exercise regimen including aerobic activity and stretching is beneficial.

When depression interferes with quality of life and activities of daily living, antidepressant therapy with a selective serotonin reuptake inhibitor (SSRI), tricyclic antidepressant or other atypical antidepressants may be added (see **Table1**).

OPTIMIZING DOPAMINERGIC TREATMENT

- Adjunct therapy with dopamine agonist may be considered.

Although rigorous clinical trial data are lacking regarding the use of SSRIs and TCAs in the treatment of depression in PD, their use is widespread in clinical practice and

Table 1
Commonly used drugs in PD depression

Drug Class/ Intervention Strategy	Drug	Dose	Side Effects	Comments
TCA MDS evidence based review: possibly useful[35]	Amitriptyline (tertiary amine)	Total daily dose: 50–200 mg/d	Significant central and peripheral antimuscarinic side effects (eg, dry mouth, blurry vision, constipation, confusion, hallucination, hypotension, sedation, sexual dysfunction, cardiac arrhythmia, seizure precipitation and weight gain)	Subset of patients with PD with drooling and bladder dysfunction, the antimuscarinic effect may be beneficial
	Imipramine (tertiary amine)	Total daily dose: 50–200 mg/d	Often undesirable and intolerable to elderly patients Arrhythmias may occur at higher concentration	Sedating TCA like amitriptyline may be beneficial in patients with insomnia
	Desipramine (Norpramin)	Total daily dose: 75 mg/d	Anticholinergic side effects, sedation	Rapid onset within 14 d
	Nortriptyline (Pamelor)	Total daily dose: 50–150 mg/d Starting dose: 10–25 mg qd Maintenance dose: 50–150 mg qd best taken HS		Less cardiac arrhythmia less antimuscarinic and CNS effects

	Drug	Dosing	Side effects	Comments
SSRI MDS evidence based review: possibly useful[35]	Citalopram (Celexa)	Total daily dose: 20–40 mg/d; Starting dose: 10–20 mg qd; Maintenance dose: 20–40 mg qd	May worsen PD tremor in ≤5% of patients and occasionally worsen parkinsonism; Fewer anticholinergic side effects, cardiac arrhythmias compared with TCAs; Nausea, dry mouth, somnolence, insomnia	No weight gain; In ≥60 y when used in a daily dose of more than 20 mg carries the risk of Corrected QT interval (QTc) prolongation; Regular monitoring electrocardiograph is recommended
	Escitalopram oxalate (Lexapro)	Starting dose: 10 mg qd Geriatric dosing of 5 mg/d; Maintenance dose: 10–20 mg qd	Nausea, insomnia, ejaculatory disorder, diarrhea	
	Fluoxetine (Prozac)	Total daily dose: 20–40 mg/d; Starting dose: 10–20 mg qd; Maintenance dose: 10–40 mg qd	Insomnia, sexual dysfunction, GI side effects	No antimuscarinic side effects, no increased risk of cardiac arrhythmia, hypotension, seizure; Less sedation; CyP 450 inhibitors: increased risk of drug interactions
	Sertraline (Zoloft)	Total daily dose: 50–150 mg/d; Starting dose: 25–50 mg qd; Maintenance dose: 50–150 mg qd	Sexual dysfunction, GI side effects, insomnia	
	Paroxetine (Paxil)[27]	Total daily dose: 20–50 mg/d; Starting dose: 10–20 mg qd; Maintenance dose: 20–40 mg qd	Sexual dysfunction, GI side effects	CyP 450 inhibitors: increased risk of drug interactions

(continued on next page)

Table 1
(continued)

Drug Class/ Intervention Strategy	Drug	Dose	Side Effects	Comments
SNRIs MDS evidence based review: Clinically useful	Venlafaxine (Effexor, Effexor XR)[27]	Total daily dose: 75–150 mg/d Starting dose: 37.5–75 mg qd Maintenance dose: 75–150 mg qd The initial starting dose is 37.5 mg/d. It should be titrated slowly up to a maximum of 150 mg/d in the elderly patient. It is also available in an extended release preparation.	Sexual dysfunction, GI side effects, insomnia	No weight gain Potential activating effect: venlafaxine (37.5–150 mg/d) should be given in the morning or early afternoon Avoid later in the day, especially in patients with insomnia or sleep disturbances Used with caution in hypertensive patients: may raise blood pressure
Dopamine agonist MDS evidence based review: Clinically useful	Pramipexole (Mirapex) mention about using with caution in the elderly	Start at 0.125 mg PO TID and titrated to a maximally tolerated dose, but no higher than 4.5 mg/d in 3 divided doses	Somnolence at a dose above 1.5 mg/d, hypotension, hallucination	Dopamine withdrawal syndrome and increased rates of apathy and depression following rapid medication reduction after deep brain stimulation surgery
MDS evidence based review: investigational	Rotigotine (Neupro)	Starting dose 2 mg/d increase as needed by 2 mg/d at weekly intervals, ≤8 mg/d	Nausea, vomiting, somnolence, application site reactions, dizziness, anorexia, hyperhidrosis, insomnia, peripheral edema, dyskinesia	

Atypical antidepressants	Mirtazipine (Remeron)	Starting dose 7.5 mg/d may increase to 30 mg/d at bedtime	Constipation, dry mouth, orthostasis, sedation, weight gain	Effective in combination with psychotherapy Oral clearance is reduced in the elderly Weight loss Sedative but no anticholinergic or arrhythmia side effects: better suited for elderly Serotonin syndrome: increased risk when coadministered with other serotonergic agents (eg, SSRI, SNRI, triptans), but also when taken alone
	Trazodone (Desyrel)	Starting dose: 150 mg in divided doses daily with food. Usually used HD starting at 50 mg maximum dose: 400 mg/d in divided doses	Priapism, mild anxiolytic, edema, blurred vision, syncope, drowsiness, fatigue, diarrhea, nasal congestion	
	Bupropion (Wellbutrin)	Starting dose: 50–100 mg qd Maintenance dose: 150–450 mg qd	Agitation, constipation, dry mouth, excessive sweating, tremor, weight loss. Uncommon side effects include seizures and psychosis at high doses.	No adverse on sexual function (as can SSRIs). No significant cardiac side effects. Potential activating effect: bupropion (50–200 mg/d) should be given in the morning CyP 450 inhibitors: Increased risk of drug interactions.
rTMS MDS evidence based review: possibly useful[35]				Concluded some beneficial effect of rTMS on depression
Cognitive-behavioral therapy MDS evidence based review: possibly useful[35]				Significant decreases in depression scores with a maintenance of the effect over the follow-up periods of 1 and 6 mo

Abbreviations: CNS, central nervous system; GI, gastrointestinal; HS, at bedtime; qd, once daily; rTMS, repetitive transcranial magnetic stimulation; SNRI, Serotonin–noradrenaline reuptake inhibitor; SSRI, Selective serotonin re-uptake inhibitors; TCA, tricyclic antidepressant; TID, 3 times a day.

generally well tolerated. Based on overall scientific data and clinical experience tricyclic antidepressant and SSRIs may be a first-line pharmacologic agent for the treatment of PD depression. Patients may benefit from an SSRI, which may be effective for both anxiety and depression, which often coexist. In cases of nonsuicidal depressed patients with severe anxiety, short-term use of benzodiazepines, such as lorazepam (0.5–1.0 mg) or clonazepam (0.5–1.0 mg) up to 2 to 3 times daily may be beneficial. Once therapeutic improvement is attained, it is advisable to keep the stable dose of medications at least for 6 months to prevent recurrence.

In patients with depression and psychotic features, initial steps involve minimizing polypharmacy and lowering dopaminergic medications as tolerated. Treatment with both an antidepressant and antipsychotic is recommended. Currently, quetiapine, an atypical antipsychotic agent, is the first-line agent, because it is well-tolerated with a low risk of extrapyramidal side effects. The usual recommended dose is 12.5 to 25 mg at bedtime. Owing to its sedating effect, quetiapine may be helpful in depressed patients with PD with insomnia or rapid eye movement sleep disorder.

Clozapine (Clozaril) may also be effective for PD psychosis. A major complication of clozapine is agranulocytosis and patients have to be regularly monitored for neutropenia. Pimavanserin, a selective serotonin 5-HT2A inverse agonist, is approved by the US Food and Drug Administration for the treatment of hallucinations and delusions associated with PD psychosis. Most common adverse reactions are peripheral edema and confusion.

NONPHARMACOLOGIC THERAPY

- Adequate sleep
- Good nutrition: Depression may be associated with anorexia.
- Regular exercise program: An exercise regimen of 20 to 30 min of aerobic activity at 60% to 70% maximum heart rate, as well as adequate stretching may be useful.
- Individual or family counseling as well as psychotherapy may be offered as an adjuvant to treatment with an antidepressant.
- Patient and caregivers should be introduced to local PD support groups and national organizations to raise awareness regarding mood disturbances in PD, ways to cope with emotional stress and obtain adequate support.
- Cognitive-behavioral therapy: A systematic review of cognitive-behavioral therapy for depression in PD found 2 randomized controlled trials. Cognitive-behavioral therapy lead to significant reductions in depression scores with a maintenance of the effect over the follow-up periods of 1 and 6 months.[28]
- Repetitive transcranial magnetic stimulation: Although there was no clear evidence of an improvement of mood symptoms when compared with sham transcranial magnetic stimulation[29,30] others concluded some beneficial effect of repetitive transcranial magnetic stimulation on depression in PD lasting at least 30 days after treatment.[31]

MANAGEMENT OF ANXIETY

- Lack of randomized clinical trials with anxiety as primary outcome.
- Anxiety is more prevalent in patients with motor fluctuations, and may worsen gait.

The first management strategy for anxiety is to reduce off periods using dopamine replacement therapy in patients with motor fluctuations, and then consider other pharmacologic interventions. The Movement Disorders Society task force found insufficient evidence to make specific recommendations for the treatment of anxiety in PD. Commonly used drugs for anxiety are discussed in **Table 2**. Devos and colleagues[32] in a placebo-controlled randomized clinical trial with desipramine (75 mg/d) and citalopram (20 mg/d) showed that anxiety scores were significantly better than the placebo group at 30 days with desipramine and citalopram. Menza and colleagues[33]

Table 2
Management of anxiety in PD

Drugs	Efficacy	Special Considerations
Lorazepam and alprazolam for short term, PRN management	Long acting benzodiazepine: improved the psychic and somatic (eg, tremor)symptom	Short-term relieve of anxiety, but the effects are gradually attenuated.
Clonazepam	Effective in anxiety and panic disorder refractory to alprazolam, lorazepam and numerous antidepressants	Increase risk of falls and fractures in older people
		Not recommended in patients with postural reflex disturbances.
		Reduced alertness, cognitive disabilities and gait disturbances
Buspirone	10–40 mg/d for a period of 12 wk has modest beneficial effect on anxiety	Higher daily doses 100 mg/d result in enhanced anxiety and worsened Parkinsonism.
	Therapeutic onset of Buspirone requires ≤6 wk to detect its anxiolytic effects	
Citalopram Sertraline Paroxetine	Anxiolytic effect in patients with PD.	Acute side effects like agitation, diarrhea, insomnia and nausea may occur.
	SSRIs are well tolerated	Occasionally SSRI may worsen tremor
		Chronic use is associated with development of endocrinology and metabolic side effects like hyponatremia, sexual dysfunction and weight gain
		The concomitant use of amantadine may reduce the risk of SSRI induced sexual dysfunction
		Increased risk of falls
		Concomitant used of MaO B inhibitors (eg, selegeline, rasageline): Increased risk of 5-HT syndrome, however the overall risk seems to be minimal
		Abrupt discontinuation may lead to withdrawal syndrome. Gradual tapering of dose recommended.
Desipramine, nortriptyline	TCAs significantly relieved anxiety compared with placebo	Adverse events are more prevalent for tricyclic antidepressants than for SSRIs

Abbreviations: 5-HT, serotonin; MaO B, monoamine oxidase B; PD, Parkinson disease; PRN, as needed; SSRI, selective serotonin reuptake inhibitor.

showed that nortriptyline significantly relieved anxiety compared with placebo, but paroxetine did not.

The pooled effect size of 4 antidepressants citalopram, desipramine, paroxetine, and nortriptyline in 2 clinical trials by Devos and colleagues[32] and Menza and colleagues[33] showed no statistical significance 1.13 (95% confidence interval, −0.67 to 2.94). However, when divided into SSRIs (citalopram and paroxetine) and tricyclic antidepressants (desipramine and nortriptyline), the effect size for tricyclic antidepressants was significant, whereas that for the SSRIs was not.[34] When anxiety is present along with depression, there may be a slow initial response to antidepressant therapy.

Outpatient Screening for Depression and Suicidality

The Patient Health Questionnaire-2 (PHQ-2) is used as initial outpatient screen for depression. If a patient scores 2 or higher on either of PHQ-2 questions, he or she is asked to complete the PHQ-9 to further evaluate depressive symptoms. If a patient answers more than half the days or nearly every day to the ninth PHQ-9 question about thoughts that you would be better off dead, or of hurting yourself in the last 2 weeks, the patient is given a brief version of the Columbia Suicide Severity Rating Scale to assess for suicidality. Patients with suicidal ideation should receive prompt treatment with antidepressants and psychiatric referral may be considered in addition to emergency room referral for active suicidal ideation.

SUMMARY

Depression and anxiety are prevalent psychiatric features in patients with PD, which contribute to accelerated disability and functional morbidity and correlate with poor quality of life and increased caregiver burden. Early detection and adequate treatment may provide substantial improvement in patients with PD. Older patients likely focus on somatic and vegetative complains of fatigue, loss of energy, pain, reduced sexual desire and functioning, and sleep disturbances, which are prominent symptoms of mood disorder as well as PD itself. Thus, symptoms of depression and anxiety in PD may be falsely attributed to features of PD and therefore go unrecognized and undetected. An individualized multimodal approach utilizing education, social support, and psychotherapeutic intervention along with pharmacologic intervention should be considered.

REFERENCES

1. Weintraub D, Moberg PJ, Duda JE, et al. Effect of psychiatric and other nonmotor symptoms on disability in Parkinson's disease. J Am Geriatr Soc 2004;52:784–8.
2. Bach J-P, Riedel O, Klotsche J, et al. Impact of complications and comorbidities on treatment costs and health-related quality of life of patients with Parkinson's disease. J Neurol Sci 2012;314(1–2):41–7.
3. Balestrino R, Martinez-Martin P. Reprint of "neuropsychiatric symptoms, behavioural disorders, and quality of life in Parkinson's disease". J Neurol Sci 2017; 374:3–8.
4. Jones JD, Butterfield LC, Song W, et al. Anxiety and depression are better correlates of Parkinson's disease quality of life than apathy. J Neuropsychiatry Clin Neurosci 2015;27(3):213–8.
5. Duncan GW, Khoo TK, Yarnall AJ, et al. Health-related quality of life in early Parkinson's disease: the impact of nonmotor symptoms. Mov Disord 2014;29(2): 195–202.

6. Fan J-Y, Chang B-L, Wu Y-R. Relationships among depression, anxiety, sleep, and quality of life in patients with Parkinson's disease in Taiwan. Parkinsons Dis 2016;2016:4040185.

7. Marsh L, McDonald WM, Cummings J, et al. Provisional diagnostic criteria for depression in Parkinson's disease: report of an NINDS/NIMH work group. Mov Disord 2006;21:148–58.

8. Weintraub D, Moberg PJ, Duda JE, et al. Recognition and treatment of depression in Parkinson's disease. J Geriatr Psychiatry Neurol 2003;16:178–83.

9. Schrag A, Ben-Shlomo Y, Quinn N. How common are complications of Parkinson's disease? J Neurol 2002;249:419–23.

10. Alonso A, Rodriguez LA, Logroscino G, et al. Use of antidepressants and the risk of Parkinson's disease: a prospective study. J Neurol Neurosurg Psychiatry 2009; 80:671–4.

11. Broen MP, Narayen NE, Kuijf ML, et al. Prevalence of anxiety in Parkinson's disease: a systematic review and meta-analysis. Mov Disord 2016;31:1125–33.

12. Chen JJ. Anxiety, depression, and psychosis in Parkinson's disease: unmet needs and treatment challenges. Neurol Clin 2004;22:S63–90.

13. Schrag A. Psychiatric aspects of Parkinson's disease—an update. J Neurol 2004; 251:795–804.

14. Walsh K, Bennett G. Parkinson's disease and anxiety. Postgrad Med J 2001;77: 89–93.

15. Menza MA, Robertson-Hoffman DE, Bonapace AS. Parkinson's disease and anxiety: comorbidity with depression. Biol Psychiatry 1993;34(7):465–70.

16. Brown RG, Landau S, Hindle JV, et al. Depression and anxiety related subtypes in Parkinson's disease. J Neurol Neurosurg Psychiatry 2011;82:803–9.

17. Burn DJ, Landau S, Hindle JV, et al. Parkinson's disease motor subtypes and mood. Mov Disord 2012;27:379–86.

18. Schrag A, Taddei RN. Depression and anxiety in Parkinson's disease. Int Rev Neurobiol 2017;133:623–55.

19. Belarbi S, Hecham N, Lesage S, et al. LRRK2 G2019S mutation in Parkinson's disease: a neuropsychological and neuropsychiatric study in a large Algerian cohort. Parkinsonism Relat Disord 2010;16:676–9.

20. Beavan M, McNeill A, Proukakis C, et al. Evolution of prodromal clinical markers of Parkinson disease in a GBA mutation-positive cohort. JAMA Neurol 2015;72: 201–8.

21. Aarsland D, Pahlhagen S, Ballard CG, et al. Depression in Parkinson disease—epidemiology, mechanisms and management. Nat Rev Neurol 2011;8:35–47.

22. Lauterbach EC, Freeman A, Vogel RL. Correlates of generalized anxiety and panic attacks in dystonia and Parkinson disease. Cogn Behav Neurol 2003;16: 225–33.

23. Miyasaki JM, Shannon K, Voon V, et al. Practice parameter: evaluation and treatment of depression, psychosis, and dementia in Parkinson disease (an evidence-based review): report of the quality standards Subcommittee of the American Academy of Neurology. Neurology 2006;66:996–1002.

24. Schrag A, Barone P, Brown RG, et al. Depression rating scales in Parkinson's disease: critique and recommendations. Mov Disord 2007;22(8):1077–92.

25. Leentjens AF, Dujardin K, Marsh L, et al. Anxiety rating scales in Parkinson's disease: critique and recommendations. Mov Disord 2008;23:2015–25.

26. Sawabini KA, Watts RL. Treatment of depression in Parkinson's disease. Parkinsonism Relat Disord 2004;10:S37–41.

27. Richard IH, McDermott MP, Kurlan R, et al, SAD-PD Study Group. A randomized, double-blind, placebo-controlled trial of antidepressants in Parkinson disease. Neurology 2012;78(16):1229–36.

28. Egan SJ, Laidlaw K, Starkstein S. Cognitive behaviour therapy for depression and anxiety in Parkinson's disease. J Parkinsons Dis 2015;5:443–51.

29. Brys M, Fox MD, Agarwal S, et al. Multifocal repetitive TMS for motor and mood symptoms of Parkinson disease: a randomized trial. Neurology 2016;87:1907–15.

30. Shin HW, Youn YC, Chung SJ, et al. Effect of high-frequency repetitive transcranial magnetic stimulation on major depressive disorder in patients with Parkinson's disease. J Neurol 2016;263:1442–8.

31. Pal E, Nagy F, Aschermann Z, et al. The impact of left prefrontal repetitive transcranial magnetic stimulation on depression in Parkinson's disease: a randomized, double-blind, placebo-controlled study. Mov Disord 2010;25:2311–7.

32. Devos D, Dujardin K, Poirot I, et al. Comparison of desipramine and citalopram treatments for depression in Parkinson's disease: a double- blind, randomized, placebo-controlled study. Mov Disord 2008;23:850–7.

33. Menza M, Dobkin RD, Marin H, et al. A controlled trial of antidepressants in patients with Parkinson disease and depression. Neurology 2009;72:886–92.

34. Troeung L, Egan SJ, Gasson N. A meta-analysis of randomized placebo controlled treatment trials for depression and anxiety in Parkinson's disease. PLoS One 2013;8:e79510.

35. Seppi K, Ray Chaudhuri K, Coelho M, et al. Update on treatments for nonmotor symptoms of Parkinson's disease—an evidence-based medicine review. Mov Disord 2019;34:180–98.

Hallucinations, Delusions and Impulse Control Disorders in Parkinson Disease

Karlo J. Lizarraga, MD, MS[a,b,c,d,e,*], Susan H. Fox, MRCP(UK), PhD[a,b,c], Antonio P. Strafella, MD, PhD[a,b,c], Anthony E. Lang, MD[a,b,c]

KEYWORDS

- Parkinson disease • Psychosis • Hallucinations • Delusions • Delirium
- Compulsions • Impulse control disorders • Dopamine dysregulation syndrome

KEY POINTS

- Psychosis and impulse control disorders (ICDs) are challenging complications in Parkinson disease.
- Delirium should be suspected when acute psychosis is associated with confusion and disorientation.
- Medications for Parkinson disease can trigger or worsen psychosis. Yet, the underlying cause is also related to Parkinson disease pathology, and often reducing or discontinuing drugs will not completely resolve psychosis.
- Management of Parkinson disease psychosis includes reduction and/or discontinuation of anticholinergics, amantadine, or dopaminergic drugs. Adjunctive therapies include cholinesterase inhibitors for visual hallucinations, the 5-HT-2A receptor inverse agonist pimavanserin, and the atypical antipsychotics quetiapine and clozapine. All other antipsychotics may worsen motor symptoms and should be avoided.
- Long-term monitoring for ICDs might lead to timely dopamine agonist discontinuation and symptom resolution. However, some patients experience disabling withdrawal symptoms.

INTRODUCTION

The 6 illustrative patients described by James Parkinson more than 200 years ago did not exhibit obvious psychiatric symptoms.[1] Although Parkinson disease (PD) is still

[a] The Edmond J. Safra Program in Parkinson Disease and the Morton and Gloria Shulman Movement Disorders Clinic, Division of Neurology, Department of Medicine, Toronto Western Hospital, University Health Network, Toronto, Ontario, Canada; [b] University of Toronto, Toronto, Ontario, Canada; [c] Krembil Research Institute, Toronto, Ontario, Canada; [d] Motor Physiology and Neuromodulation Program, Division of Movement Disorders, Department of Neurology, University of Rochester, Rochester, New York, United States; [e] Center for Health + Technology (CHeT), University of Rochester, Rochester, New York, United States
* Corresponding author. 399 Bathurst Street, McL 7-412, Toronto, Ontario, M5T 2S8, Canada.
E-mail address: karlo.lizarraga@gmail.com

Clin Geriatr Med 36 (2020) 105–118
https://doi.org/10.1016/j.cger.2019.09.004
0749-0690/20/© 2019 Elsevier Inc. All rights reserved.
geriatric.theclinics.com

considered a movement disorder, the introduction of effective therapies for motor symptoms over the past 60 years and the increasing lifespan of patients have allowed for the recognition of neuropsychiatric symptoms as being highly prevalent, disabling, and associated with poor outcomes and quality of life.[2]

The incidence of Parkinson disease increases exponentially with age.[3] When Parkinson disease begins at older ages, nonmotor symptoms appear earlier, and aging further exacerbates neuropsychiatric complications of Parkinson disease.[4] Despite their frequent occurrence and association with adverse outcomes, these symptoms are not yet fully understood and are still under-recognized and undertreated in Parkinson disease.[5]

The most common neuropsychiatric symptoms in Parkinson disease are cognitive dysfunction, depression, and psychosis. Compulsive symptoms, including impulse control disorders (ICDs), are also relatively common in Parkinson disease, although more common in younger patients. This article provides practical recommendations to diagnose and manage psychotic and compulsive disturbances in Parkinson disease.

APPROACH TO COMPULSIVE AND PSYCHOTIC SYMPTOMS IN PARKINSON DISEASE
Compulsive Symptoms

In Parkinson disease, hypersensitivity to reward and a hyperdopaminergic state might lead to compulsive symptoms associated with impulsivity. These include ICDs, dopamine dysregulation syndrome (DDRS), hobbyism and more rarely hoarding (**Table 1**).[6] ICDs are repetitive, reward-seeking, uncontrollable behaviors (behavioral addictions) leading to impaired functioning and quality of life. It is paramount to regularly monitor patients for the development of ICDs and recognize them in a timely fashion, as they might profoundly affect patients and caregivers, resulting in poor personal, financial, social, and health outcomes.

Younger patients with Parkinson disease might develop punding, which is usually associated with excessive and intense preoccupation with items or activities, and can be induced by high doses of antiparkinsonian medications. DDRS (associated with behaviors characteristic of drug addiction) typically manifests in younger male patients who usually have minimal motor symptoms but usually have dyskinesia and take dopaminergic medications despite being in a pronounced dyskinetic state. Punding and DDRS share the repetitive and excessive compulsive features and relationship with hyperdopaminergic state.

Psychotic Symptoms

Hallucinations and delusions are the most common psychotic manifestations in Parkinson disease. In addition, the clinical spectrum of Parkinson disease psychosis includes illusions and minor phenomena such as presence and passage. According to the criteria for PD psychosis from the National Institute of Neurologic Disorders and Stroke/National Institute of Mental Health (NINDS/NIMH), the diagnosis requires at least 1 of the following: illusions, false sense of presence or passage, hallucinations, or delusions. These features should occur after Parkinson disease onset and be present for at least 1 month, either as recurrent or continuous symptoms. Acute delirium and other medical, neurologic, or psychiatric causes should be excluded.[7]

Hallucinations

In Parkinson disease, these misperceptions are frequently visual, clear, vivid and with similar impact as normal perceptions. Visual hallucinations in PD range from

Table 1	
Common compulsive, misperception and delusional symptoms	
Compulsive Symptom	**Abnormal Behavior**
Obsession	Intrusive repetitive thoughts, urges, images, or impulses that trigger anxiety and that the patient is unable to suppress
Compulsion	Repetitive behavior or mental act responding to obsession or done according to rigid rules intended to reduce distress caused by obsessions
Punding	Complex, prolonged, purposeless, stereotyped behavior usually experienced as comforting but of which interruption can result in anger (eg, disassembling and reassembling objects, rearranging papers)
Dopamine dysregulation syndrome	Addictive-like regimen of self-medicating with high doses of dopaminergic medications, particularly the short-acting dopamine agonist apomorphine and levodopa
Hoarding	Excessive accumulation of belongings unrelated to their value and difficulty discarding them due to associated anxiety and need to save
Misperception Symptom	**Abnormal Perception**
Illusion	Misperception of existent sensory stimulus
Hallucination	Misperception without external sensory stimulus
Palinopsia	Persistent visual stimulus after that stimulus is no longer present
Synesthesia	Stimulus perceived outside sensory modality in which it is presented or adding features not normally perceived within a sensory modality
Derealization	Perceiving/experiencing the external world as unreal
Depersonalization	Perceiving/experiencing oneself as detached from one's mental processes of body (as if an outside observer)
Autoscopy	Seeing one's body from a position outside the body
Déjà vu	Perceiving/experiencing a novel image or scene as one previously witnessed or experienced
Deja entendu	Perceiving/experiencing a novel sound as one previously witnessed or experienced
Jamais vu	Perceiving/experiencing a familiar image or scene as unfamiliar
Jamais entendu	Perceiving/experiencing a familiar sound as unfamiliar
Delusional Symptom	**Abnormal Belief or Delusional Misidentification**
Delusion	Fixed belief not amenable to change in light of conflicting evidence
Othello	Delusional jealousy-belief that the spouse (usually the wife of a male patient) is having an extramarital affair
Capgras	Spouse or other familiar individual replaced by an impostor who is physically but not psychologically identical to the replaced person
Frégoli	Different people are in fact a single person (usually believed to be a persecutor) who changes appearance or is in disguise

(continued on next page)

Table 1 (continued)	
Delusional Symptom	**Abnormal Belief or Delusional Misidentification**
Intermetamorphosis (Variant of Frégoli)	Familiar people and strangers in the environment swap identities while maintaining their original appearance
Subjective doubles	Double of oneself exists, carrying out independent actions (also known as subjective Capgras delusion)
Clonal pluralization	Multiple physically and psychologically identical copies of oneself
Delusional companions	Nonliving objects are sentient beings
Mirrored self-misidentification	One's reflection in a mirror is someone else
Reduplicative paramnesia	A familiar person, place, or object has been duplicated
Cotard	One or more of one's organs or body parts missing or no longer existing

nonformed to clearly defined visions taking human, animal, or object shapes (eg, mice scurrying on the floor, children playing in the house). Many of them are nonthreatening and brief, but become worse at night or when vision is compromised. In particular, alterations in visual acuity are an acknowledged risk factor for visual hallucinations in Parkinson disease.

Nonvisual hallucinations are now recognized as relatively common in Parkinson disease.[8] As opposed to primary psychiatric conditions, auditory hallucinations in Parkinson disease are usually less defined and less likely to be threatening, derogatory, commanding, or directly interact with the patient. Of note, musical hallucinations necessitate audiologic evaluation, as hypoacusis is the most common cause.[9] Tactile, olfactory, and gustatory hallucinations are unusual, and their presence suggests other causes. Nonvisual hallucinations are frequently accompanied by their visual counterparts and occur more frequently in advanced Parkinson disease. There is a higher risk for chronicity and recurrence once multimodal hallucinations are simultaneously present.[10]

Other perceptual disturbances considered psychotic in earlier Parkinson disease include the interpretation of inanimate objects as living beings (different from delusional companion syndrome) (see **Table 1**). Presence hallucinations evoke the false sense that someone is nearby, whereas passage hallucinations involve the sensation of a person or animal passing in the peripheral visual field. These latter 2 symptoms are especially common in Parkinson disease and do not forewarn of the development of more severe formed visual hallucinations.

Hallucinations should be distinguished from other perceptual phenomena that are not necessarily pathologic (see **Table 1**), especially if they occur with preserved insight and are not associated with other neuropsychiatric disturbances or functional decline. Hallucinations that occur while falling asleep (hypnagogic) or waking up (hypnapompic) may be a symptom of narcolepsy, but they are considered within the normal range of experience. Interestingly, some hallucinations in Parkinson disease might represent narcolepsy-like manifestations of rapid eye movement (REM) sleep behavior disorder (RBD). Theoretically, either short REM latency when falling asleep or continuation of REM into partial wakefulness might be associated with hallucinations having particular characteristics such as frequent vision of human figures or faces, animals, or scenery of great beauty.[11]

Delusions

These fixed beliefs are often divided into ordinary and bizarre. Ordinary delusions are more common in Parkinson disease. They derive from misinterpretation of everyday experiences and, as such, are possible but not acceptable. Bizarre delusions are more common in primary psychosis and involve phenomena that are physically impossible or at least implausible.

In Parkinson disease, delusions are less frequent than hallucinations and affect 5% to 10% of patients.[8] The most common type of delusions in Parkinson disease are persecutory, involving a belief that someone is monitoring or trying to harm the patient. When questioned about these beliefs, patients will not be able to reason through any explanations. Often, the person trying to help the patient will become part of the delusions. Other common themes include jealousy, spousal infidelity, and paranoia. In contrast, reference and grandiose delusions are more common in primary psychotic disorders.

Delusional misidentification syndromes are frequent in Parkinson disease dementia but might be encountered in Parkinson disease with only mild cognitive impairment (see **Table 1**). These delusions are associated with impairments in facial processing, and although they may occur in psychiatric illness, as many as 20% to 40% arise in the context of neurologic conditions affecting the right hemisphere.[12]

DELIRIUM IN PARKINSON DISEASE

Delirium is an acute and fluctuating impairment in attention and awareness accompanied by cognitive dysfunction in the setting of a systemic insult. Delirium in Parkinson disease may be underdiagnosed, because its circadian, behavioral and perceptive disturbances, including delusions and hallucinations, overlap with chronic neuropsychiatric manifestations and/or dopaminergic side effects. Thus, acute and/or episodic confusion and disorientation might be more specific for delirium in Parkinson disease. Notably, confusional states at night time or upon arousing from sleep in patients with Parkinson disease might be associated with RBD.[11]

Management

Table 2 summarizes the suggested management of delirium in Parkinson disease.

After timely recognition, systemic comorbidities and precipitating factors should be treated and prevented.[13] Some triggering factors that might occur in Parkinson disease are reduced fluid intake and dehydration caused by dysphagia and anticholinergic-induced urinary retention. Afterward, the indications to continue unnecessary and potentially harmful drugs need to be revised.[14] As a rule of thumb, drugs with least dopaminergic and most anticholinergic effects should be withdrawn first. In many cases, reducing polypharmacy and tapering dopaminergic medication doses might be successful. However, patients with Parkinson disease might not tolerate dopaminergic medication reductions and require compensatory levodopa increases to prevent severe akinetic-rigid symptoms. It should be kept in mind that stopping amantadine, anticholinergics, dopamine agonists (DAs), and levodopa has been associated with severe and even fatal withdrawal syndromes.[15]

The use of psychoactive medications during delirium in patients with Parkinson disease should be carefully considered only to palliate severe agitation, psychosis, or anxiety. Neuroleptics are commonly used, but all typical and most atypical antipsychotics are contraindicated in these patients because of the risk of significantly worsening parkinsonism. In fact, most systematic studies have evaluated neuroleptics for

Table 2
Suggested management of delirium in Parkinson disease

Treatment	Examples	Comments/Adverse Effects
Step 1 Identify and treat systemic illnesses, avoid causative and precipitating factors	• Infections • Opioids • Benzodiazepines • Anticholinergics • Steroids	Avoid/prevent: quinolones, cefepime, opioids, dehydration (dysphagia), urinary retention (anticholinergics, dysautonomia), untreated pain
Step 2 Reduce and/or discontinue potentially harmful or unnecessary medications	• Anticholinergics (urologic, trihexyphenidyl) • Antidepressants (tricyclics) • Analgesics (opioids) • Antibiotics (quinolones, cefepime)	Tapering recommended instead of abrupt withdrawal of anticholinergics
Step 3 Nonpharmacological measures (sensory, emotional, and environmental support)	• Reorientation • Visual and hearing aids • Support sleep-wake cycle • Early mobilization • Translation services • Maintain contact with familiar persons	Avoid/prevent: sleep deprivation, dehydration, poor nutrition, sensory deprivation, physical restraints, unstable and/or uncomfortable environment (eg, room changes, noise), aspiration, falls
Step 4 Reduce doses of dopaminergic medications as needed (suggested order based on anticholinergic/dopaminergic effects)	1. Anticholinergics 2. Amantadine 3. MAO-B inhibitors 4. Dopamine agonists 5. COMT inhibitors 6. Levodopa	Tapering recommended instead of abrupt withdrawal (except for selegiline and other MAO-B inhibitors)
Step 5 Symptom management: • Worsening parkinsonism • Sleep-wake cycle disturbances • Night-time confusion and early morning hallucinations caused by RBD • Severe psychosis and/or agitation (monitor for conversion of hyperactive to hypoactive delirium).	• Adjust levodopa dose to account for Step 4 (crush and administer via nasogastric tube if needed) • Melatonin: 2–12 mg taken 1–2 h before bedtime • Clonazepam: 0.5–1 mg QHS • Quetiapine: Start at 25 mg/d (preferably QHS) and gradually increase up to 150 mg/d as needed • Clozapine: Start at 6.25, 12.5 or 25 mg/d and gradually increase up to 100 mg/d as needed	• Levodopa: agitation, confusion, psychosis • Melatonin: not proven effective but safe • Clonazepam: sedation • Quetiapine: possibly safe–monitor for hypotension, sedation, sialorrhea, worsening of parkinsonism • Clozapine: possibly safe but often avoided Monitor for same as quetiapine plus seizures, hyperglycemia in diabetics, metabolic syndrome, myocarditis, venous thromboembolism, drug interactions, agranulocytosis Central anticholinergic effects at higher doses might worsen delirium

Abbreviations: COMT, Catechol-O-methyltransferase; MAO-B, monoamine oxidase B; QHS, from Latin "quaque hora somni" (every bedtime); RBD, rapid eye movement sleep behavior disorder.

chronic hallucinations but not for delirium in Parkinson disease.[5,16,17] As will be discussed in the next section, quetiapine if often favored over clozapine.

There are no studies on the use of acetylcholinesterase inhibitors or benzodiazepines for delirium in Parkinson disease. However, rivastigmine has been associated with longer delirium duration and mortality.[18] Other drugs such as melatonin and low-dose clonazepam might be cautiously used when significant RBD symptoms are present. In fact, melatonin has been associated with decreased incidence of delirium in hospitalized elderly patients.[19]

CHRONIC PSYCHOSIS IN PARKINSON DISEASE

Recent research suggests a prevalence of 42% for minor hallucinations in newly diagnosed, untreated Parkinson disease patients.[20] When the NINDS/NIMH criteria were applied to a cross-sectional Parkinson disease cohort, prevalence was 60%, compared with 43% when defined only by hallucinations and/or delusions.[8] Additionally, a prospective study encompassing Parkinson disease patients on dopaminergic treatment reported long-term cumulative prevalence of 60%.[21]

Psychosis in Parkinson disease is associated with poor quality of life, worse prognosis, and caregiver stress.[22] Psychosis is the greatest risk factor for nursing home placement, major cause of recurrent hospitalizations, and an independent predictor of increased mortality in patients with Parkinson disease.[23,24]

Potential risk factors for psychosis in Parkinson disease include older age, polypharmacy, axial rigidity, and cognitive impairment.[25,26] Parkinson disease patients with psychosis exhibit greater cognitive deficits, particularly in attention, executive, and visuospatial abilities. Moreover, most of them report disturbances of sleep and wakefulness, including RBD.[27]

Hallucinations occur more frequently with DAs than with levodopa.[28] In particular, age greater than 65 years is a significant risk factor for hallucinations associated with pramipexole.[29] Despite the association between drug exposure and psychosis in Parkinson disease, the dosage and duration of treatment do not clearly correlate with psychosis.[25] In fact, high-dose intravenous levodopa does not seem to precipitate hallucinations in Parkinson disease patients with pre-existing hallucinations.[30]

Management

Fig. 1 depicts a proposed algorithm for the management of chronic Parkinson disease psychosis.

Many psychotic symptoms in Parkinson disease are brief, nonthreatening, and not bothersome for patients or caregivers. For instance, some patients report pleasant hallucinations such as lonely nursing home residents who enjoy observing playful children. Thus, careful observation with management of comorbid conditions and discontinuation or reduction of nonessential medications may be sufficient for many patients, at least in the short term.[13]

Psychosis may improve with dopaminergic dose reduction or cessation. Although there is no high-quality evidence to support this strategy, Parkinson disease medications are usually reduced sequentially and gradually.[31] Of note, switching dopaminergic therapy to apomorphine infusion for other indications has been associated with reduced psychosis.[32] Antagonism of the 5-HT-2A serotonin receptor and/or D1-receptor activation by apomorphine may explain the lower risk of hallucinations with this drug.[33]

After baseline QT interval is obtained through electrocardiogram (ECG), acetylcholinesterase inhibitors may also reduce visual hallucinations in Parkinson disease

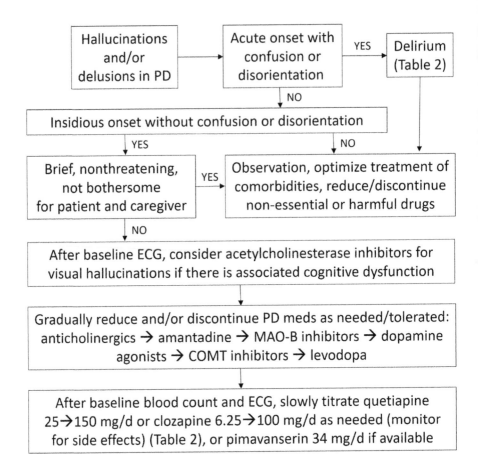

Fig. 1. Proposed algorithm for the management of psychosis in Parkinson disease. COMT, Catechol-O-methyltransferase; MAO-B, monoamine oxidase B; PD, Parkinson disease.

patients with cognitive dysfunction. Because donepezil has been associated with heightened arousal, it should be administered in the morning in order to avoid night-time insomnia.[34]

Co-administration of quetiapine or clozapine might be needed for bothersome psychosis when dopaminergic drugs cannot be reduced without worsening parkinsonism. ECG monitoring for QT interval prolongation is also required upon initiation of these drugs, particularly in older patients.[35,36]

As demonstrated in clinical trials, low-dose clozapine (25–50 mg/d) is efficacious for Parkinson disease psychosis without worsening motor function.[16,17,37] Yet, this drug is rarely used likely because of required blood monitoring for potential granulocytopenia and agranulocytosis.[38] When clozapine is initiated, patients are usually enrolled in a hematological monitoring program able to prevent or reverse most of these cases.

Clozapine-induced granulocytopenia is dose-dependent and occurs in approximately 1% of patients. Agranulocytosis has occurred only in 0.38% of patients in a large sample of schizophrenia patients in the United States.[39] There are no data in Parkinson disease, but the risk is probably smaller given the considerably lower doses used. For instance, the authors have not observed any case of agranulocytosis in the Parkinson disease patients on chronic clozapine therapy followed at the Toronto Western Hospital.[40]

Other adverse events with clozapine include sedation, orthostatic hypotension, sialorrhea, myocarditis, venous thromboembolic events including pulmonary embolism, and significant drug interactions (see **Table 2**). Importantly, clozapine has central anticholinergic properties at higher doses that might worsen RBD and delirium. Of note, clozapine appears to have antidystonic, antidyskinetic, and even antitremor effects that might be beneficial in Parkinson disease.[40]

Although the evidence favors clozapine, quetiapine is the most commonly used atypical antipsychotic in patients with Parkinson disease. Quetiapine demonstrated comparable efficacy to clozapine and relatively low risk of adverse effects in observational studies. Yet, controlled trials with reasonable sample sizes have been negative or hard to interpret.[41–43]

Pimavanserin is a selective serotonin-2A receptor inverse agonist without dopamine receptor-blocking properties. This novel agent was US Food and Drug Administration (FDA) approved in 2016 for Parkinson disease psychosis on the basis of a single randomized controlled trial (RCT) because of breakthrough therapy designation.[44] Given recent controversies regarding the primary outcome measure used in this RCT, the possibly delayed onset, and questions about mortality, additional research is needed to confirm the efficacy and safety of pimavanserin, particularly in Parkinson disease patients with comorbid dementia.[45] Another challenge is its high cost and lack of availability outside of the United States.

As previously mentioned, typical and other atypical antipsychotics should be avoided because of the risk of worsening Parkinson disease motor symptoms.[46] Recent studies have suggested increased morbidity and mortality for Parkinson disease patients on antipsychotics,[47] similar to Alzheimer disease patients, for whom all antipsychotics carry a black box warning.

IMPULSE CONTROL DISORDERS IN PARKINSON DISEASE

The increased recognition of compulsive behaviors in Parkinson disease patients over the last 15 years coincides with the introduction and use of D2-D3 receptor-selective DAs. Initial studies showed that ICDs occur relatively commonly in treated Parkinson disease patients.[48] More recent studies have confirmed that ICD rates are not elevated in de novo, untreated patients compared with age-matched controls.[49] In the largest cross-sectional study to date, ICDs were identified in 13.6% of treated Parkinson disease patients (5.7% compulsive buying, 5% gambling, 4.3% binge eating, and 3.5% compulsive sexual behavior). Moreover, 29% of these patients had more than one ICD.[50] A recent multisite study reported a 5-year cumulative ICD incidence rate of 46%, although this study recruited patients before significant changes were made in DA prescribing.[51] Another study found clinically significant ICDs in 36% of treated Parkinson disease patients with dyskinesias.[52]

ICDs remain generally under-recognized, because patients may not report such behaviors due to embarrassment, lack of suspicion of the association with Parkinson disease drugs, or unwillingness to stop the causative drug or the ICD itself. In fact, patient reporting is often discrepant from that of other informants.[53]

DA treatment is the strongest factor associated with ICDs in Parkinson disease (17.1% taking DA vs 6.9% not taking DA).[50,51] ICDs appear to be a drug class adverse effect, as no significant differences exist among the different DAs, except for reduced risk with apomorphine infusion. The initial reports of potentially reduced ICD risk with long-acting DAs such as rotigotine patch[54] were not confirmed in a recent larger study.[51]

ICD development may be associated with higher dose and longer duration of DA exposure. Thus, ongoing long-term vigilance is required, because ICDs may not begin until many years after DA initiation.[55] DA effects do not appear unique to patients with Parkinson disease, as similar associations with ICDs have been reported (eg, in restless legs syndrome on lower doses of DA), and thus there may not be a dose-related risk.[56]

Higher-dose levodopa, amantadine, and monoamine oxidase B inhibitors have also been associated with ICDs in Parkinson disease, although to a lesser extent compared with DAs and usually in subjects on multiple drugs.[50,57] Intrinsic factors associated with ICDs in Parkinson disease are age and gender. ICDs are more likely to occur in younger male patients and less likely with later Parkinson disease onset, though male gender remains a risk factor in older patients.[58] Unmarried status, personal or family history of substance abuse, gambling, impulsive or novelty-seeking behavior, depression, and anxiety have emerged as potential additional factors.[48,50,59] Therefore, it is important to inquire and document these features in patients with Parkinson disease, particularly before initiating DA therapy. The nature of the ICD is more likely to be sexual in men as opposed to buying and binge eating in women.[6]

DDRS and other compulsive disorders in PD tend to occur with higher doses of levodopa. For example, a large study reported less than 2% frequency of punding in patients with Parkinson disease, which increased to 14% when Parkinson disease patients on higher doses of levodopa were studied.[60,61] The short-acting subcutaneous injections of apomorphine, used as rescue therapy during unpredictable off periods, might also be abused in a similar fashion as levodopa.[62]

Management

ICDs/DDRS and compulsive symptoms are typically more responsive to reducing/stopping the offending agent. ICDs typically improve and resolve after DA reduction.[63] However, some patients might not tolerate DA reduction or discontinuation. In fact, a DA withdrawal syndrome with dysphoria, anxiety, pain, and cravings has been described 15% to 20% of these patients.[15] Worsening of motor and/or neuropsychiatric symptoms might require compensatory increases of other dopaminergic drugs and even consideration of advanced therapies such as continuous levodopa-carbidopa intestinal infusion.[64] As for individuals with gambling and other behavioral addictions unrelated to Parkinson disease, patients with Parkinson disease under observation/treatment for ICDs would also benefit from support systems able to monitor symptoms and limit access to or completely avoid triggers.

Although there is not enough evidence to support their use, other medications have been employed to treat ICDs in patients with Parkinson disease (eg, antidepressants, antipsychotics, mood stabilizers, and donepezil). For example, a small RCT reported amantadine as beneficial for pathologic gambling in patients with Parkinson disease, but as previously noted, amantadine has been associated with ICDs in a larger epidemiologic study.[57,65] DDRS is far more challenging to manage, as patients resist reducing addictive use of high-dose levodopa, and collaboration with psychiatry colleagues is often required.

SUMMARY

The prevalence of neuropsychiatric complications in Parkinson disease is high and associated with worse outcomes, impaired quality of life, and greater caregiver burden. Psychotic and compulsive symptoms in Parkinson disease are frequently iatrogenic given their relationship with dopaminergic therapy, particularly DAs. Upon acute presentation, delirium should be ruled out and treated accordingly (see **Table 2**). For chronic symptoms, comorbid systemic illnesses, substance abuse, dementia, and primary psychiatric disorders should be kept in mind. Careful reduction and discontinuation of anticholinergic and dopaminergic medications, as well as adjunctive therapy with clozapine or quetiapine, is usually successful for the management of Parkinson disease psychosis (see **Fig. 1**). Pimavanserin is a novel agent for which more experience is required. ICDs require frequent monitoring, documentation, and caregiver involvement, as timely DA discontinuation is usually successful. Large epidemiologic, genetic, and neurobiological studies are needed to inform future trials to establish more efficacious and better-tolerated therapies for psychosis and ICDs in Parkinson disease.

REFERENCES

1. Obeso JA, Stamelou M, Goetz CG, et al. Past, present, and future of Parkinson's disease: a special essay on the 200th anniversary of the shaking palsy. Mov Disord 2017;32:1264–310.
2. Weintraub D, Burn D. Parkinson's disease: the quintessential neuropsychiatric disorder. Mov Disord 2011;26:1022–31.
3. Marras C, Beck JC, Bower JH, et al. Prevalence of Parkinson's disease across North America. NPJ Parkinsons Dis 2018;4:21.
4. Levy G. The relationship of Parkinson disease with aging. Arch Neurol 2007;64:1242–6.
5. Seppi K, Ray Chaudhuri K, Coelho M, et al. Update on treatments of nonmotor symptoms of Parkinson's disease-an evidence-based medicine review. Mov Disord 2019;34:180–98.
6. Weintraub D, David AS, Evans EH, et al. Clinical spectrum of impulse control disorders in Parkinson's disease. Mov Disord 2015;30:121–7.
7. Ravina B, Marder K, Fernandez HH, et al. Diagnostic criteria for psychosis in Parkinson's disease: report of an NINDS, NIMH work group. Mov Disord 2007;22:1061–8.
8. Fenelon G, Soulas T, Zenasni F, et al. The changing face of Parkinson's disease-associated psychosis: a cross-sectional study based on the new NINDS-NIMH criteria. Mov Disord 2010;25:763–6.
9. Coebergh JA, Lauw RF, Bots R, et al. Musical hallucinations: review of treatment effects. Front Psychol 2015;6:814.
10. Goetz CG, Stebbins GT, Ouyang B. Visual plus nonvisual hallucinations in Parkinson's disease: development and evolution over 10 years. Mov Disord 2011;26:2196–200.
11. Arnulf I, Bonnet A-M, Damier P, et al. Hallucinations, REM sleep, and Parkinson's disease: a medical hypothesis. Neurology 2000;55:281–8.
12. Christodoulou GN, Margariti M, Kontaxakis VP, et al. The delusional misidentification syndromes: strange, fascinating, and instructive. Curr Psychiatry Rep 2009;11:185–9.
13. Thomsen TR, Panisset M, Suchowersky O, et al. Impact of standard of care for psychosis in Parkinson disease. J Neurol Neurosurg Psychiatry 2008;79:1413–5.
14. Rudolph JL, Salow MJ, Angelini MC, et al. The anticholinergic risk scale and anticholinergic adverse effects in older persons. Arch Intern Med 2008;168:508–13.

15. Rabinak C, Nirenberg M. Dopamine agonist withdrawal syndrome in Parkinson disease. Arch Neurol 2010;67:58–63.
16. Parkinson Study Group. Low-dose clozapine for the treatment of drug-induced psychosis in Parkinson's disease. N Engl J Med 1999;340:757–63.
17. Pollak P, Tison F, Rascol O, et al. Clozapine in drug induced psychosis in Parkinson's disease: a randomized, placebo controlled study with open follow up. J Neurol Neurosurg Psychiatry 2004;75:689–95.
18. van Eijk MM, Roes KC, Honing ML, et al. Effect of rivastigmine as an adjunct to usual care with haloperidol on duration of delirium and mortality in critically ill patients: a multicenter, double-blind, placebo-controlled randomized trial. Lancet 2010;376:1829–37.
19. Chen S, Shi L, Liang F, et al. Exogenous melatonin for delirium prevention: a meta-analysis of randomized controlled trials. Mol Neurobiol 2016;53:4046–53.
20. Pagonabarraga J, Martinez-Horta S, Fernandez de Bobadilla R, et al. Minor hallucinations occur in drug-naive Parkinson's disease patients, even from the premotor phase. Mov Disord 2016;31:45–52.
21. Forsaa E, Larsen J, Wentzel-Larsen T, et al. A 12-year population-based study of psychosis in Parkinson disease. Arch Neurol 2010;67:996–1001.
22. McKinlay A, Grace R, Dalrymple-Alford J, et al. A profile of neuropsychiatric problems and their relationship to quality of life for Parkinson's disease patients without dementia. Parkinsonism Relat Disord 2008;14:37–42.
23. Forsaa E, Larsen J, Wentzel-Larsen T, et al. What predicts mortality in Parkinson disease? A prospective population-based long-term study. Neurology 2010;75: 1270–6.
24. Factor S, Feustel P, Freidman J, et al. Longitudinal outcome of Parkinson's disease patients with psychosis. Neurology 2003;60:1756–61.
25. Aarsland D, Larsen J, Cummings J, et al. Prevalence and clinical correlates of psychotic symptoms in Parkinson disease: a community-based study. Arch Neurol 1999;56:595–601.
26. Marsh L, Williams J, Rocco M, et al. Psychiatric comorbidities in patients with Parkinson disease and psychosis. Neurology 2004;63:293–300.
27. Pacchetti C, Manni R, Zangaglia R, et al. Relationship between hallucinations, delusions, and rapid eye movement sleep behavior disorder in Parkinson's disease. Mov Disord 2005;20:1439–48.
28. Rascol O, Brooks DJ, Korczyn AD, et al. A five-year study of the incidence of dyskinesia in patients with early Parkinson's disease who were treated with ropinirole or levodopa. N Engl J Med 2000;342:1484–91.
29. Parkinson Study Group CALM Cohort Investigators. Long-term effect of initiating pramipexole vs. levodopa in early Parkinson disease. Arch Neurol 2009;66: 563–70.
30. Goetz CG, Pappert EJ, Blasucci LM, et al. Intravenous levodopa in hallucinating Parkinson's disease patients: high-dose challenge does not precipitate hallucinations. Neurology 1998;50:515–7.
31. Olanow C, Stern M, Sethi K. The scientific and clinical basis of the treatment of Parkinson disease. Neurology 2009;72(21 suppl 4):S1–136.
32. Borgemeester RW, Lees AJ, van Laar T. Parkinson's disease, visual hallucinations and apomorphine: a review of the available evidence. Parkinsonism Relat Disord 2016;27:35–40.
33. Manson AJ, Hanagasi H, Turner K, et al. Intravenous apomorphine therapy in Parkinson's disease: clinical and pharmacokinetic observations. Brain 2001;124(Pt 2):331–40.

34. Bergman J, Lerner V. Successful use of donepezil for the treatment of psychotic symptoms in patients with Parkinson's disease. Clin Neuropharmacol 2002;25: 107–10.
35. Alvir JM, Lieberman JA, Safferman AZ, et al. Clozapine-induced agranulocytosis. Incidence and risk factors in the United States. N Engl J Med 1993;329:162–7.
36. Shah AA, Aftab A, Coverdale J. QTc prolongation with antipsychotics: is routine ECG monitoring recommended? J Psychiatr Pract 2014;20:196–206.
37. The French Clozapine Parkinson Study Group. Clozapine in drug-induced psychosis in Parkinson's disease. Lancet 1999;353:2041–2.
38. Weintraub D, Chen P, Ignacio R, et al. Patterns and trends in antipsychotic prescribing for Parkinson disease psychosis. Arch Neurol 2011;68:899–904.
39. Honigfeld G, Arellano F, Sethi J, et al. Reducing clozapine-related morbidity and mortality: 5 years of experience with the Clozaril National Registry. J Clin Psychiatry 1998;59(Suppl 3):3–7.
40. Yaw TK, Fox SH, Lang AE. Clozapine in Parkinsonian rest tremor: a review of outcomes, adverse reactions, and possible mechanisms of action. Mov Disord Clin Pract 2015;3:116–24.
41. Ondo W, Tintner R, Voung K, et al. Double-blind, placebo-controlled, unforced titration parallel trial of quetiapine for dopaminergic-induced hallucinations in Parkinson's disease. Mov Disord 2005;20:958–63.
42. Rabey J, Prokhorov T, Miniovitz A, et al. Effect of quetiapine in psychotic Parkinson's disease patients: a double-blind labeled study of 3 months' duration. Mov Disord 2007;22:313–8.
43. Shotbolt P, Samuel M, Fox C, et al. A randomized controlled trial of quetiapine for psychosis in Parkinson's disease. Neuropsychiatr Dis Treat 2009;5:327–32.
44. Cummings J, Isaacson S, Mills R, et al. Pimavanserin for patients with Parkinson's disease psychosis: a randomized, placebo-controlled phase 3 trial. Lancet 2014; 383:533–40.
45. Schubmehl S, Sussman J. Perspective on pimavanserin and the SASP-PD: novel scale development as a means to FDA approval. Am J Geriatr Psychiatry 2018; 26:1007–11.
46. Friedman JH, Factor SA. Atypical antipsychotics in the treatment of drug-induced psychosis in Parkinson's disease. Mov Disord 2000;15:201–11.
47. Weintraub D, Chiang C, Kim HM, et al. Association of antipsychotic use with mortality risk in patients with Parkinson disease. JAMA Neurol 2016;73:535–41.
48. Voon V, Fox S. Medication-related impulse control and repetitive behaviors in Parkinson disease. Arch Neurol 2007;64:1089–96.
49. Weintraub D, Papay K, Siderowf A, et al. Screening for impulse control disorder symptoms in patients with de novo Parkinson disease: a case-control study. Neurology 2013;80:176–80.
50. Weintraub D, Koester J, Potenza M, et al. Impulse control disorders in Parkinson disease: a cross-sectional study of 3090 patients. Arch Neurol 2010;67:589–95.
51. Corvol JC, Artaud F, Cormier-Dequaire F, et al. Longitudinal analysis of impulse control disorders in Parkinson disease. Neurology 2018;91:e189–201.
52. Biundo R, Weis L, Abbruzzese G, et al. Impulse control disorders in advanced Parkinson's disease with dyskinesia: the ALTHEA study. Mov Disord 2017;32: 1557–65.
53. Papay K, Mamikonyan E, Siderowf A, et al. Patient versus informant reporting ICD symptoms in Parkinson's disease using the QUIP: validity and variability. Parkinsonism Relat Disord 2011;17:153–5.

54. Rizos A, Sauerbier A, Antonini A, et al. A European multicentre survey of impulse control behaviours in Parkinson's disease patients treated with short- and long-acting dopamine agonists. Eur J Neurol 2016;23:1255–61.

55. Bastiaens J, Dorfman BJ, Christos PJ, et al. Prospective cohort study of impulse control disorders in Parkinson's disease. Mov Disord 2013;28:327–33.

56. Cornelius J, Tippmann-Peikert M, Slocumb N, et al. Impulse control disorders with the use of dopaminergic agents in restless legs syndrome: a case-control study. Sleep 2010;33:81–7.

57. Weintraub D, Sohr M, Potenza M, et al. Amantadine use associated with impulse control disorders in Parkinson disease in cross-sectional study. Ann Neurol 2010; 68:963–8.

58. Carriere N, Kreisler A, Dujardin K, et al. Impulse control disorders in Parkinson's disease: a cohort of 35 patients. Rev Neurol (Paris) 2012;168:143–51.

59. Voon V, Sohr M, Lang A, et al. Impulse control disorders in Parkinson disease: a multicenter case-control study. Ann Neurol 2011;69:986–96.

60. Miyasaki J, Hassan K, Lang A, et al. Punding prevalence in Parkinson's disease. Mov Disord 2007;22:1179–81.

61. Evans A, Katzenschlager R, Paviour D, et al. Punding in Parkinson's disease: its relation to the dopamine dysregulation syndrome. Mov Disord 2004;19:397–405.

62. Cilia R, Siri C, Canesi M, et al. Dopamine dysregulation syndrome in Parkinson's disease: from clinical and neuropsychological characterization to management and long-term outcome. J Neurol Neurosurg Psychiatry 2014;85:311–8.

63. Mamikonyan E, Siderowf A, Duda J, et al. Long-term follow-up of impulse control disorders in Parkinson's disease. Mov Disord 2008;23:75–80.

64. Martinez-Martin P, Reddy P, Katzenschlager R, et al. EuroInf: a multicenter comparative observational study of apomorphine and levodopa infusion in Parkinson's disease. Mov Disord 2015;30:510–6.

65. Thomas A, Bonnani L, Gambi F, et al. Pathological gambling in Parkinson disease is reduced by amantadine. Ann Neurol 2010;68:400–4.

Overview of Sleep and Circadian Rhythm Disorders in Parkinson Disease

Priti Gros, MD[a],*, Aleksandar Videnovic, MD, MSc[b]

KEYWORDS

- Parkinson disease • Sleep disorders • Insomnia • Somnolence • RLS • RBD
- Circadian rhythm disorders • Nonmotor symptoms

KEY POINTS

- Sleep disorders are among the most common nonmotor symptoms of Parkinson disease (PD), can occur at any stage of the disease, and significantly affect quality of life.
- This article provides an overview of different sleep disorders affecting patients with PD, including insomnia, excessive daytime sleepiness, sleep-disordered breathing, restless legs syndrome, circadian rhythms disorders, and rapid eye movement sleep behavior disorders.
- Nonpharmacologic and pharmacologic treatment options are used in the management of disorders of sleep in PD.
- Further research on the pathophysiology and treatment of sleep dysfunction associated with PD is needed.

INTRODUCTION

Parkinson disease (PD) is the second most common neurodegenerative disease. Up to 98% of patients with PD report experiencing at least 1 nonmotor symptom (NMS),[1,2] among which sleep disorders are some of the most common. NMSs are underreported and underrecognized by patients with PD, caregivers, and health care providers.[2] Common barriers to seeking help include acceptance of symptoms, lack of awareness that a symptom is associated with PD, and belief that no treatments are available.[2]

Disclosure: The authors have nothing to disclose.
Conflicts of Interests: The authors declare that they have no conflicts of interest.
Funding: The authors acknowledge research support from NIH/NINDS. Grant number: R01NS099055.
[a] Division of Neurology, University of Toronto, St. Michael's Hospital, 30 Bond Street, 3 Shuter, Office 3-040, Toronto, Ontario M5B 1W8, Canada; [b] Movement Disorders Unit, Division of Sleep Medicine, Massachusetts General Hospital, Harvard Medical School, Neurological Clinical Research Institute, 165 Cambridge Street, Suite 600, Boston, MA 02114, USA
* Corresponding author.
E-mail address: priti.gros@mail.utoronto.ca

In a cross-sectional survey of 358 patients with PD, up to 30% of patients with PD failed to report sleep disorders to their health care providers[2]; their prevalence can be as high as 40% in other studies.[1] Sleep disorders are associated with significant quality-of-life impairment.[3] Further interventions need to be put in place to encourage patients with PD to report sleep disorders. Moreover, greater awareness about common sleep disorders in PD among health care providers can potentially lead to timely diagnosis and appropriate treatment.

This article discusses common sleep problems in PD, including insomnia, excessive daytime sleepiness (EDS), sleep-disordered breathing (including obstructive sleep apnea [OSA]), restless legs syndrome (RLS), circadian rhythm disorders, and rapid eye movement (REM) sleep behavior disorders (RBDs).

MOST COMMON SLEEP DISORDERS ASSOCIATED WITH PARKINSON DISEASE
Insomnia

Definition
Insomnia is the persistent difficulty to initiate, maintain, and consolidate sleep or to generate an overall good sleep quality, despite satisfying opportunity for sleep and resulting in daytime impairment.[4] Patients with PD more often report sleep fragmentation and early awakenings, rather than sleep initiation difficulty.[5]

Epidemiology
Insomnia is thought to be the most common sleep disorder in PD, with its prevalence varying from 30% to 80%.[6,7] With disease progression, the sleep maintenance problem increases in prevalence.[6]

Pathophysiology
The elements contributing to insomnia in PD are multiple. Insomnia in PD seems to be associated with PD duration and depression.[5,6] The sleep regulatory centers and circadian rhythm circuits are affected by the neurodegenerative process.[8] Moreover, patients with PD are commonly affected by multiple symptoms, such as nocturnal hypokinesia, dystonia, pain, mood changes, and nocturia, which can impair sleep.[9,10] Dopaminergic agents also have an impact on sleep, although their exact effects on various PD stages, including issues of timing and dosing of these medications, remain to be clarified.[5]

Diagnosis
A thorough sleep history, including a sleep log and the bed partner's perspective, is necessary. Questionnaires can be helpful to capture night sleep disturbances and daytime impairments.[11] Multiple questionnaires have been validated in PD, among which the PD Sleep Scale (PDSS) and its second version PDSS-II, the Scale for Outcomes in PD (SCOPA) sleep scale have been the most commonly used.[12] Polysomnography should be considered if comorbid sleep disorders are suspected.

Clinical implications
Insomnia and depression are closely related, with one often coexisting with the other.[5] Patients with PD with insomnia tend to have more advanced PD and it is often associated with balance problems (known as postural instability) and gait difficulties, frequent wearing off of the levodopa effect, autonomic dysfunction, and hallucinations.[5,13] Another element to consider is the concomitant presence of other sleep disorders, such as OSA, RBD, and RLS, which can contribute to sleep fragmentation and overall poor sleep. Insomnia and poor sleep quality are associated with lower health-related quality of life.[14]

Management

The first step in managing insomnia in PD is to review possible contributors. Patients with PD should be evaluated for potential nocturnal motor symptoms. Controlled-release levodopa or a dopamine agonist can be considered. One such agonist, trans-dermal rotigotine patch, has the advantage of providing a stable plasma level for 24 hours[15] and has been shown to help with subjective sleepiness and sleep architecture.[16,17]

The most recent evidence-based medicine update on treatment of NMSs authored by Seppi and colleagues[18] concluded that eszopiclone and melatonin are possibly useful for treatment of insomnia in PD. Nonpharmacologic circadian-based interventions such as light therapy are noninvasive feasible options for treatment of insomnia in PD.[19]

Mood disorders should be screened and treated. Venlafaxine, tricyclic antidepressants, cognitive-behavior therapy, and even the dopamine agonist pramipexole have good evidence for their use for mood disorders in PD.[18]

Excessive Daytime Sleepiness

Definition

EDS is the difficulty to remain awake and alert during the day, which leads to unintended episodes of sleep or drowsiness.[4] Sleep attacks can occur in patients with EDS and are defined by unintended and inappropriate episodes of falling sleep with minimal or no prodrome of drowsiness.[4]

Epidemiology

The prevalence of EDS in PD ranges from 20% to 75%.[20,21] A multicenter longitudinal study showed similar prevalence of EDS in untreated patients with PD compared with healthy controls[22]; however, EDS increased in prevalence over time in PD, whereas it remained unchanged among controls.

Pathophysiology

Multiple factors are associated with EDS in PD, such as PD stage, comorbid sleep disorders, and use of dopaminergic agents. Liguori and colleagues[23] suggested that EDS can occur independently of other sleep-wake disorders, possibly because neurodegeneration affects regions such as the hypothalamus and various brainstem nuclei responsible for sleep-wake regulation.[24] Dopaminergic drugs have been associated with EDS and sleep attacks, dopamine agonists being the most frequent offending agents.[25] Dopaminergic drugs possibly have a dose-related effect on EDS.[22]

Diagnosis

The Epworth Sleepiness Scale (ESS) is a commonly used screening tool. Certain electrophysiologic tests are the gold standard and they include the Multiple Sleep Latency Test (MSLT) and the Maintenance of Wakefulness Test.[26] Comorbid sleep disorders such as RLS, OSA, and RBD may influence EDS and therefore should be screened or tested with polysomnography.

Clinical implications

EDS is associated with older age, advanced PD stage, presence of postural instability and gait disturbance, autonomic dysfunction, and mood disorders.[20,27,28] EDS is also associated with worse motor function, cognitive impairment, and worse quality of life. Several studies revealed dissociation between the degree of daytime sleepiness and quality of nocturnal sleep; this raises a possibility for differential effects of PD-specific neurodegeneration on wake-promoting vs sleep regulatory centers.

Management

Management of EDS requires identifying possible reversible causes. Decreasing or discontinuing dopamine agonists,[25] as well as treating OSA, RLS, or RBD if present, can improve EDS.[29,30] Timed light therapy showed a significant improvement in ESS score in a randomized placebo-controlled study.[31] Seppi and colleagues[18] concluded that modafinil was possibly useful for treatment of EDS. Caffeine is currently investigational because there is insufficient evidence.[18] A recent study for the use of sodium oxybate in treating EDS showed significant improvement of ESS and MSLT. However, the study sample was small and long-term polysomnographic monitoring is necessary to assess treatment-related complications.[32] It is a controlled drug with special requirements that is best left to be managed by sleep specialists.

Sleep-Related Breathing Disorders

Definition

Sleep-related breathing disorders (SBDs) include OSA, central sleep apnea, sleep-related hypoventilation, and sleep-related hypoxemia. In PD, OSA is the most common form of SBD.

Epidemiology

The prevalence of OSA in PD is from 20% to 60%.[33,34] There is a significant variability in study methodologies, including scoring system used by different sleep laboratories.[35] For example, 3 different standard hypopnea definitions lead to important scoring differences and therefore differences in the estimations of OSA prevalence in the general population.[36] Further understanding of the mechanism of OSA in PD is necessary to better interpret potential scoring biases.[35]

Pathophysiology

High body mass index is typically associated with higher risk of OSA in the general population,[37] but is not associated with the severity of the OSA in PD.[38] This finding suggests that the mechanism of OSA may be different in PD. Upper airway obstruction in PD, such as laryngopharyngeal motor dysfunction, has been reported as a possible mechanism of OSA.[39] Certain studies have reported responsiveness of OSA to levodopa.[40,41]

Diagnosis

Polysomnography or home sleep apnea testing is recommended for the diagnosis of sleep apnea in the general population.[42] In PD, home sleep apnea testing has been validated in 1 study with a level III portable monitoring.[43] It had a reasonable specificity for moderate to severe OSA and therefore was considered suitable to rule in OSA but not to rule it out.[43]

Clinical implications

OSA is associated with EDS and cognitive dysfunction.[44] RBD is associated with less severe OSA in PD, possibly because of the increased motor activity during REM sleep.[45] However, patients with PD with RBD and OSA have worse cognitive dysfunction.[45]

Management

Seppi and colleagues[18] concluded that continuous positive airway pressure (CPAP) is likely efficacious and possibly useful in improving sleep and daytime sleepiness. Prolonged CPAP treatment improved anxiety, cognitive function, and overall sleep quality after 12 months of CPAP use.[30] An alternative to CPAP, such as carbidopa/levodopa (controlled-release formulation) at bedtime possibly improves OSA in PD.[40]

Restless Legs Syndrome

Definition

RLS is the urge to move the legs, usually associated with leg discomfort.[4] By definition, the latter must be caused or exacerbated by inactivity and be at least partially relieved by movement. Symptoms start or worsen in the evening or night, and cause significant discomfort.[4] RLS is closely associated with periodic limb movement of sleep (PLMS), which usually are simple stereotyped movements that can also be associated with nocturnal or diurnal disturbance.[4]

Epidemiology

A meta-analysis found that the prevalence of RLS is 14% in PD, slightly higher in patients who previously received PD treatment (15%) compared with drug-naive patients (11%).[46] RLS is associated with an increased risk of incident PD (0.37% of PD incidence in the RLS population vs 0.13% in the controls).[47] Lee and colleagues[48] suggested that the development of RLS in PD was associated with the duration of antiparkinsonian therapy. In a similar vein, other investigators have reported a lack of association between untreated PD and RLS.[49] Other studies suggest that patients with PD with RLS have older age at PD onset, more advanced PD stages, severe limb parkinsonism, depression, anxiety, dysautonomia, and worse nutritional status.[50,51]

Pathophysiology

Ferini-Strambi and colleagues[52] recently reviewed the literature around 3 main pathophysiologic hypotheses: (1) given the common responsiveness to dopaminergic therapy, RLS and PD may share a common dopaminergic pathophysiology as well as possible genetic links[53]; (2) RLS in PD may have a different mechanism than idiopathic RLS; and (3) RLS and PD may be 2 different diseases.[52] Therefore, the interaction between RLS and PD has not been settled.

In addition, there is evidence of a link between RLS and diminished iron stores in many RLS cases (with or without concomitant PD).[54,55]

Diagnosis

The criteria required to diagnose RLS are described by the third edition of the International Classification of Sleep Disorders (ICSD-3).[4] RLS has multiple mimics, including non-PD conditions such as myalgia, leg cramps, and arthritis. These conditions need to be excluded by the clinician. Concomitant PD-related leg symptoms such as limb stiffness and dystonia may also mimic RLS.[56]

Clinical implications

RLS may be the underlying cause of insomnia, such as difficulty in sleep initiation. In addition, RLS is commonly associated with PLMS and as a consequence it can also affect sleep maintenance, can worsen sleep quality, negatively affect mood, and be associated with poor quality of life.

Management

The presence of a low serum ferritin level and search for medications potentially responsible for RLS exacerbation should be assessed.[54] Evidence-based recommendations suggest dopamine agonists including pramipexole,[57] rotigotine,[58] ropinirole[59] as well as nondopaminergic options such as gabapentin enacarbil,[60] pregabalin,[61] and intravenous iron.[55] However, dopamine agonists can lead to augmentation (requirement of ever-increasing doses) or worsening of symptoms after a transient period of amelioration.[55] In such cases, dopamine agonists may be suspended or transitioned to a long-acting dopaminergic or nondopaminergic agent.[62] Subthalamic nucleus deep brain stimulation may improve RLS in PD.[63,64]

Circadian Rhythm Disorders

Circadian rhythm disorders are characterized by a chronic or recurrent sleep disturbance caused by alteration of the circadian system or a misalignment between the endogenous circadian rhythm and socially determined sleep-wake schedules.[4] PD itself is influenced by the circadian rhythm. Patients with PD may experience diurnal fluctuations in motor and nonmotor symptoms despite stable pharmacokinetics of dopaminergic medications. They may also experience seasonal fluctuations as their disease progresses.[65,66]

Mechanisms underlying these fluctuations remain unclear. Neurodegeneration affects central structures responsible for the regulation of sleep and wakefulness. PD-specific changes may affect input to the hypothalamic suprachiasmatic nucleus (SCN), the central pacemaker of the circadian system. For example, reduced exposure to ambient light and the degeneration of dopamine-containing cells in the retina of patients with PD may negatively affect the input to the SCN that is needed for alignment of dark/light cycles. Dopaminergic therapy has a possible bidirectional influence on the circadian rhythm.[67]

Light is the main zeitgeber (time giver) for the SCN, and may also have a direct alerting effect.[68] In PD, light therapy improves daytime sleepiness, sleep fragmentation, sleep quality, ease of falling asleep, and mood.[31] Furthermore, some studies even suggest light therapy has a positive effect on motor function in PD.[69]

The use of chronotherapeutics in PD, including timed bright light, physical exercise, and melatonin, is the subject of ongoing research. These therapies have the potential to be available, inexpensive, and noninvasive.[70] Further studies will be necessary to optimize PD tailored protocols.[54]

Rapid Eye Movement Sleep Behavior Disorder

Definition
RBD is a parasomnia described as repeated sleep-related vocalization and/or complex motor behaviors during REM sleep. Polysomnography reveals that the normal loss of muscle tone during REM sleep is lost (loss of muscle atonia).[4] Patients often appear to be acting out their dreams.[4]

Epidemiology
A meta-analysis estimated the prevalence of RBD in PD at 23.6% and 3.4% in the general population.[71] Similarly, the De Novo Parkinson Cohort (DeNoPa) cohort reported the prevalence of RBD as 25% in subjects with PD compared with 2% in healthy controls.[72] Idiopathic RBD (iRBD) is considered a strong prodrome of synucleinopathies (PD and other related disorders). A recent large multicentre study reported a phenoconversion rate (non–PD-affected individuals transitioning to PD) of 6.3% per year and 73.5% after 12 years' follow-up.[73] RBD precedes the onset of parkinsonism by a median time of 13 years,[74] but may do so as far as 50 years in advance.[75]

Pathophysiology
RBD has been related to a pontomedullary dysfunction of structures that regulate REM sleep, including the locus coeruleus/subcoeruleus complex.[76]

Diagnosis
Screening questionnaires are available, including the RBD Sleep Behavior Disorder Screening Questionnaire.[77] Given the prevalence of RBD mimics, polysomnography

with electromyographic analysis is the gold standard.[78] The ICSD-3 criteria include repeated observed episodes of sleep-related vocalization and/or complex motor behaviors occurring during dream mentation, leading the patient to report dream enactment.[4] There should be a clinical suspicion or electrophysiologic confirmation that these behaviors occur during REM sleep[4] or polysomnographic evidence of REM sleep without atonia.[4] Other causes for the symptoms should be excluded, such as another sleep or psychiatric disorder, or substance or medication use.[4]

Clinical implications
When comorbid with PD, RBD is associated with a poorer prognosis for the PD. There is higher risk of more severe motor dysfunction, hallucinations, cognitive impairment, and autonomic dysfunction.[79,80] Given its strong association with PD and related disorders, counseling selected patients with iRBD (with soft neurodegenerative signs and >50 years old) about the potential risk of neurodegeneration may be considered.[81]

Management
The most important first step in managing RBD is counseling patients and their bedpartners about bedroom safety.[82] Potential causing, or aggravating, agents should be reassessed, including antidepressants.[83] Mimics such as severe OSA should be screened and treated.[82] There are no level 1 efficacy data to date for the treatment of RBD in PD. Melatonin and clonazepam have both shown efficacy in several studies.[84,85]

SUMMARY

PD is associated with multiple sleep disorders, which are common and significantly impair quality of life. Routine inquiry about sleep problems from health care providers can increase its detection and clinical management. Sleep disorders have unique considerations in PD and are reviewed in this article. Further research should focus on improving screening and diagnostic tools in the PD population. Mechanisms-oriented and patient-centered therapeutic plans should be further developed. Level 1 efficacy data for treatment of most sleep disorders in PD are still lacking.

REFERENCES

1. Chaudhuri KR, Martinez-Martin P, Schapira AH, et al. International multicenter pilot study of the first comprehensive self-completed nonmotor symptoms questionnaire for Parkinson's disease: the NMSQuest study. Mov Disord 2006;21(7): 916–23.
2. Hurt CS, Rixon L, Chaudhuri KR, et al. Barriers to reporting non-motor symptoms to health-care providers in people with Parkinson's. Parkinsonism Relat Disord 2019;64:220–5.
3. Karlsen KH, Larsen JP, Tandberg E, et al. Influence of clinical and demographic variables on quality of life in patients with Parkinson's disease. J Neurol Neurosurg Psychiatry 1999;66(4):431–5.
4. American Academy of Sleep Medicine. The international classification of sleep disorders: diagnostic and coding manual. 3rd edition. Darien (IL): American Academy of Sleep Medicine; 2014.
5. Zhu K, van Hilten JJ, Marinus J. The course of insomnia in Parkinson's disease. Parkinsonism Relat Disord 2016;33:51–7.
6. Tholfsen LK, Larsen JP, Schulz J, et al. Changes in insomnia subtypes in early Parkinson disease. Neurology 2017;88(4):352–8.

7. Loddo G, Calandra-Buonaura G, Sambati L, et al. The treatment of sleep disorders in Parkinson's disease: from research to clinical practice. Front Neurol 2017;8:42.

8. Diederich NJ, Vaillant M, Mancuso G, et al. Progressive sleep 'destructuring' in Parkinson's disease. A polysomnographic study in 46 patients. Sleep Med 2005;6(4):313–8.

9. Louter M, van Sloun RJ, Pevernagie DA, et al. Subjectively impaired bed mobility in Parkinson disease affects sleep efficiency. Sleep Med 2013;14(7):668–74.

10. Gomez-Esteban JC, Zarranz JJ, Lezcano E, et al. Sleep complaints and their relation with drug treatment in patients suffering from Parkinson's disease. Mov Disord 2006;21(7):983–8.

11. Schutte-Rodin S, Broch L, Buysse D, et al. Clinical guideline for the evaluation and management of chronic insomnia in adults. J Clin Sleep Med 2008;4(5):487–504.

12. Hogl B, Arnulf I, Comella C, et al. Scales to assess sleep impairment in Parkinson's disease: critique and recommendations. Mov Disord 2010;25(16):2704–16.

13. Chung S, Bohnen NI, Albin RL, et al. Insomnia and sleepiness in Parkinson disease: associations with symptoms and comorbidities. J Clin Sleep Med 2013;9(11):1131–7.

14. Shafazand S, Wallace DM, Arheart KL, et al. Insomnia, sleep quality, and quality of life in mild to moderate Parkinson's disease. Ann Am Thorac Soc 2017;14(3):412–9.

15. Wang HT, Wang L, He Y, et al. Rotigotine transdermal patch for the treatment of neuropsychiatric symptoms in Parkinson's disease: a meta-analysis of randomized placebo-controlled trials. J Neurol Sci 2018;393:31–8.

16. Pierantozzi M, Placidi F, Liguori C, et al. Rotigotine may improve sleep architecture in Parkinson's disease: a double-blind, randomized, placebo-controlled polysomnographic study. Sleep Med 2016;21:140–4.

17. De Fabregues O, Ferre A, Romero O, et al. Sleep quality and levodopa intestinal gel infusion in Parkinson's disease: a pilot study. Parkinsons Dis 2018;2018:8691495.

18. Seppi K, Ray Chaudhuri K, Coelho M, et al. Update on treatments for nonmotor symptoms of Parkinson's disease-an evidence-based medicine review. Mov Disord 2019;34(2):180–98.

19. Martino JK, Freelance CB, Willis GL. The effect of light exposure on insomnia and nocturnal movement in Parkinson's disease: an open label, retrospective, longitudinal study. Sleep Med 2018;44:24–31.

20. O'Suilleabhain PE, Dewey RB Jr. Contributions of dopaminergic drugs and disease severity to daytime sleepiness in Parkinson disease. Arch Neurol 2002;59(6):986–9.

21. Suzuki K, Okuma Y, Uchiyama T, et al. Impact of sleep-related symptoms on clinical motor subtypes and disability in Parkinson's disease: a multicentre cross-sectional study. J Neurol Neurosurg Psychiatry 2017;88(11):953–9.

22. Amara AW, Chahine LM, Caspell-Garcia C, et al. Longitudinal assessment of excessive daytime sleepiness in early Parkinson's disease. J Neurol Neurosurg Psychiatry 2017;88(8):653–62.

23. Liguori C, Mercuri NB, Albanese M, et al. Daytime sleepiness may be an independent symptom unrelated to sleep quality in Parkinson's disease. J Neurol 2019;266(3):636–41.

24. Braak H, Del Tredici K, Rub U, et al. Staging of brain pathology related to sporadic Parkinson's disease. Neurobiol Aging 2003;24(2):197–211.

25. Yeung EYH, Cavanna AE. Sleep attacks in patients with Parkinson's disease on dopaminergic medications: a systematic review. Movement Disord Clin Pract 2014;1(4):307–16.

26. Johns MW. Sensitivity and specificity of the multiple sleep latency test (MSLT), the maintenance of wakefulness test and the epworth sleepiness scale: failure of the MSLT as a gold standard. J Sleep Res 2000;9(1):5–11.

27. Junho BT, Kummer A, Cardoso F, et al. Clinical predictors of excessive daytime sleepiness in patients with Parkinson's disease. J Clin Neurol (Seoul, Korea) 2018;14(4):530–6.

28. Xiang YQ, Xu Q, Sun QY, et al. Clinical features and correlates of excessive daytime sleepiness in Parkinson's disease. Front Neurol 2019;10:121.

29. Neikrug AB, Liu L, Avanzino JA, et al. Continuous positive airway pressure improves sleep and daytime sleepiness in patients with Parkinson disease and sleep apnea. Sleep 2014;37(1):177–85.

30. Kaminska M, Mery VP, Lafontaine AL, et al. Change in cognition and other nonmotor symptoms with obstructive sleep apnea treatment in Parkinson disease. J Clin Sleep Med 2018;14(5):819–28.

31. Videnovic A, Klerman EB, Wang W, et al. Timed light therapy for sleep and daytime sleepiness associated with Parkinson disease: a randomized clinical trial. JAMA Neurol 2017;74(4):411–8.

32. Buchele F, Hackius M, Schreglmann SR, et al. Sodium oxybate for excessive daytime sleepiness and sleep disturbance in Parkinson disease: a randomized clinical trial. JAMA Neurol 2018;75(1):114–8.

33. Valko PO, Hauser S, Sommerauer M, et al. Observations on sleep-disordered breathing in idiopathic Parkinson's disease. PLoS One 2014;9(6):e100828.

34. Beland SG, Postuma RB, Latreille V, et al. Observational study of the relation between Parkinson's disease and sleep apnea. J Parkinsons Dis 2015;5(4):805–11.

35. Kaminska M, Lafontaine AL, Kimoff RJ. The interaction between obstructive sleep apnea and Parkinson's disease: possible mechanisms and Implications for cognitive function. Parkinsons Dis 2015;2015:849472.

36. Hirotsu C, Haba-Rubio J, Andries D, et al. Effect of three hypopnea scoring criteria on OSA prevalence and associated comorbidities in the general population. J Clin Sleep Med 2019;15(2):183–94.

37. Levy P, Kohler M, McNicholas WT, et al. Obstructive sleep apnoea syndrome. Nat Rev Dis Primers 2015;1:15015.

38. Trotti LM, Bliwise DL. No increased risk of obstructive sleep apnea in Parkinson's disease. Mov Disord 2010;25(13):2246–9.

39. Bahia C, Pereira JS, Lopes AJ. Laryngopharyngeal motor dysfunction and obstructive sleep apnea in Parkinson's disease. Sleep Breath 2019;23(2):543–50.

40. Gros P, Mery VP, Lafontaine AL, et al. Obstructive sleep apnea in Parkinson's disease patients: effect of Sinemet CR taken at bedtime. Sleep Breath 2016;20(1):205–12.

41. Tsai CC, Wu MN, Liou LM, et al. Levodopa reverse stridor and prevent subsequent endotracheal intubation in Parkinson disease patients with bilateral vocal cord palsy: a case report. Medicine (Baltimore) 2016;95(50):e5559.

42. Kapur VK, Auckley DH, Chowdhuri S, et al. Clinical practice guideline for diagnostic testing for adult obstructive sleep apnea: an American academy of sleep medicine clinical practice guideline. J Clin Sleep Med 2017;13(3):479–504.

43. Gros P, Mery VP, Lafontaine AL, et al. Diagnosis of obstructive sleep apnea in Parkinson's disease patients: is unattended portable monitoring a suitable tool? Parkinsons Dis 2015;2015:258418.

44. Mery VP, Gros P, Lafontaine AL, et al. Reduced cognitive function in patients with Parkinson disease and obstructive sleep apnea. Neurology 2017;88(12):1120–8.
45. Huang JY, Zhang JR, Shen Y, et al. Effect of rapid eye movement sleep behavior disorder on obstructive sleep apnea severity and cognition of Parkinson's disease patients. Chin Med J (Engl) 2018;131(8):899–906.
46. Yang X, Liu B, Shen H, et al. Prevalence of restless legs syndrome in Parkinson's disease: a systematic review and meta-analysis of observational studies. Sleep Med 2018;43:40–6.
47. Szatmari S Jr, Bereczki D, Fornadi K, et al. Association of restless legs syndrome with incident Parkinson's disease. Sleep 2017;40(2).
48. Lee JE, Shin HW, Kim KS, et al. Factors contributing to the development of restless legs syndrome in patients with Parkinson disease. Mov Disord 2009;24(4): 579–82.
49. Angelini M, Negrotti A, Marchesi E, et al. A study of the prevalence of restless legs syndrome in previously untreated Parkinson's disease patients: absence of co-morbid association. J Neurol Sci 2011;310(1–2):286–8.
50. Moccia M, Erro R, Picillo M, et al. A four-year longitudinal study on restless legs syndrome in Parkinson disease. Sleep 2016;39(2):405–12.
51. Fereshtehnejad SM, Shafieesabet M, Shahidi GA, et al. Restless legs syndrome in patients with Parkinson's disease: a comparative study on prevalence, clinical characteristics, quality of life and nutritional status. Acta Neurol Scand 2015; 131(4):211–8.
52. Ferini-Strambi L, Carli G, Casoni F, et al. Restless legs syndrome and Parkinson disease: a causal relationship between the two disorders? Front Neurol 2018; 9:551.
53. Alonso-Navarro H, Garcia-Martin E, Agundez JAG, et al. Association between restless legs syndrome and other movement disorders. Neurology 2019;92(20): 948–64.
54. Videnovic A. Disturbances of sleep and alertness in Parkinson's disease. Curr Neurol Neurosci Rep 2018;18(6):29.
55. Garcia-Borreguero D, Silber MH, Winkelman JW, et al. Guidelines for the first-line treatment of restless legs syndrome/Willis-Ekbom disease, prevention and treatment of dopaminergic augmentation: a combined task force of the IRLSSG, EURLSSG, and the RLS-foundation. Sleep Med 2016;21:1–11.
56. Hogl B, Stefani A. Restless legs syndrome and periodic leg movements in patients with movement disorders: specific considerations. Mov Disord 2017; 32(5):669–81.
57. Ma JF, Wan Q, Hu XY, et al. Efficacy and safety of pramipexole in Chinese patients with restless legs syndrome: results from a multi-center, randomized, double-blind, placebo-controlled trial. Sleep Med 2012;13(1):58–63.
58. Oertel WH, Benes H, Garcia-Borreguero D, et al. Rotigotine transdermal patch in moderate to severe idiopathic restless legs syndrome: a randomized, placebo-controlled polysomnographic study. Sleep Med 2010;11(9):848–56.
59. Walters AS, Ondo WG, Dreykluft T, et al. Ropinirole is effective in the treatment of restless legs syndrome. TREAT RLS 2: a 12-week, double-blind, randomized, parallel-group, placebo-controlled study. Mov Disord 2004;19(12):1414–23.
60. Walters AS, Ondo WG, Kushida CA, et al. Gabapentin enacarbil in restless legs syndrome: a phase 2b, 2-week, randomized, double-blind, placebo-controlled trial. Clin Neuropharmacol 2009;32(6):311–20.
61. Allen RP, Chen C, Garcia-Borreguero D, et al. Comparison of pregabalin with pramipexole for restless legs syndrome. N Engl J Med 2014;370(7):621–31.

62. Winkelman JW, Armstrong MJ, Allen RP, et al. Practice guideline summary: treatment of restless legs syndrome in adults: report of the guideline development, dissemination, and implementation subcommittee of the American Academy of Neurology. Neurology 2016;87(24):2585–93.
63. Chahine LM, Ahmed A, Sun Z. Effects of STN DBS for Parkinson's disease on restless legs syndrome and other sleep-related measures. Parkinsonism Relat Disord 2011;17(3):208–11.
64. Klepitskaya O, Liu Y, Sharma S, et al. Deep brain stimulation improves restless legs syndrome in patients with Parkinson disease. Neurology 2018;91(11): e1013–21.
65. Bonuccelli U, Del Dotto P, Lucetti C, et al. Diurnal motor variations to repeated doses of levodopa in Parkinson's disease. Clin Neuropharmacol 2000;23(1): 28–33.
66. Niwa F, Kuriyama N, Nakagawa M, et al. Circadian rhythm of rest activity and autonomic nervous system activity at different stages in Parkinson's disease. Auton Neurosci 2011;165(2):195–200.
67. Bolitho SJ, Naismith SL, Rajaratnam SM, et al. Disturbances in melatonin secretion and circadian sleep-wake regulation in Parkinson disease. Sleep Med 2014; 15(3):342–7.
68. Videnovic A, Messinis L. Enlightened PD: a novel treatment for Parkinson disease? Neurology 2019;92(11):499–500.
69. Willis GL, Turner EJ. Primary and secondary features of Parkinson's disease improve with strategic exposure to bright light: a case series study. Chronobiol Int 2007;24(3):521–37.
70. Fifel K, Videnovic A. Chronotherapies for Parkinson's disease. Prog Neurobiol 2019;174:16–27.
71. Zhang J, Xu CY, Liu J. Meta-analysis on the prevalence of REM sleep behavior disorder symptoms in Parkinson's disease. BMC Neurol 2017;17(1):23.
72. Mollenhauer B, Trautmann E, Sixel-Doring F, et al. Nonmotor and diagnostic findings in subjects with de novo Parkinson disease of the DeNoPa cohort. Neurology 2013;81(14):1226–34.
73. Postuma RB, Iranzo A, Hu M, et al. Risk and predictors of dementia and parkinsonism in idiopathic REM sleep behaviour disorder: a multicentre study. Brain 2019;142(3):744–59.
74. Postuma RB, Berg D. Advances in markers of prodromal Parkinson disease. Nat Rev Neurol 2016;12(11):622–34.
75. Claassen DO, Josephs KA, Ahlskog JE, et al. REM sleep behavior disorder preceding other aspects of synucleinopathies by up to half a century. Neurology 2010;75(6):494–9.
76. Boeve BF, Silber MH, Saper CB, et al. Pathophysiology of REM sleep behaviour disorder and relevance to neurodegenerative disease. Brain 2007;130(Pt 11): 2770–88.
77. Stiasny-Kolster K, Mayer G, Schafer S, et al. The REM sleep behavior disorder screening questionnaire–a new diagnostic instrument. Mov Disord 2007;22(16): 2386–93.
78. Li K, Li SH, Su W, et al. Diagnostic accuracy of REM sleep behaviour disorder screening questionnaire: a meta-analysis. Neurol Sci 2017;38(6):1039–46.
79. Kim Y, Kim YE, Park EO, et al. REM sleep behavior disorder portends poor prognosis in Parkinson's disease: a systematic review. J Clin Neurosci 2018;47:6–13.
80. St Louis EK, Boeve BF. REM sleep behavior disorder: diagnosis, clinical implications, and future directions. Mayo Clin Proc 2017;92(11):1723–36.

81. Arnaldi D, Antelmi E, St Louis EK, et al. Idiopathic REM sleep behavior disorder and neurodegenerative risk: to tell or not to tell to the patient? How to minimize the risk? Sleep Med Rev 2017;36:82–95.

82. Dauvilliers Y, Schenck CH, Postuma RB, et al. REM sleep behaviour disorder. Nat Rev Dis Primers 2018;4(1):19.

83. Gagnon JF, Postuma RB, Montplaisir J. Update on the pharmacology of REM sleep behavior disorder. Neurology 2006;67(5):742–7.

84. Aurora RN, Zak RS, Maganti RK, et al. Best practice guide for the treatment of REM sleep behavior disorder (RBD). J Clin Sleep Med 2010;6(1):85–95.

85. McCarter SJ, Boswell CL, St Louis EK, et al. Treatment outcomes in REM sleep behavior disorder. Sleep Med 2013;14(3):237–42.

Orthopedic Care of Patients with Parkinson Disease

Marian Livingston Dale, MD, MCR

KEYWORDS

- Parkinson disease • Orthopedics • Surgery • Shoulder • Spine • Hip • Knee

KEY POINTS

- Patients with Parkinson disease (PD) are at particular risk for anterior-superior dislocation of the shoulder related to supraspinatus tendon tearing and rigidity of shoulder girdle muscles.
- The chance of complications from lumbar spinal surgeries in patients with PD increases with fusion length.
- Constrained prosthetic designs, such as cruciate-retaining, condylar-constrained kinetic, or hinged devices, are recommended for patients with PD undergoing knee surgeries.

INTRODUCTION

Orthopedic complaints are common in patients with Parkinson disease (PD), but may be undertreated. In a case-control study Kim and colleagues,[1] 400 patients with PD were interviewed about their shoulder, lumbar, and knee problems. Compared with age-matched and sex-matched controls, the overall prevalence of orthopedic complaints in patients with PD was higher (66.3% vs 45.7%), but pharmacologic treatment of those complaints was less (36.7% vs 53.1%). This study excluded patients with PD with severe cognitive problems, so the extent of undertreatment may be even more than reported in this study.

This article summarizes existing literature examining orthopedic interventions for patients with PD and causes of fall-related fractures in PD. It reviews complications and functional outcomes of shoulder, spine, knee, and hip surgeries in PD. The risk of postoperative cognitive decline after orthopedic interventions in patients with PD is also briefly discussed.

CAUSES OF FALL-RELATED FRACTURES IN PARKINSON DISEASE

Fall-related fractures are common in PD. In a study of 100 patients with PD, Cheng and colleagues[2] noted that 56 patients had falls during the study period and 32 of those

Disclosure: The author has nothing to disclose.
Department of Neurology, Oregon Health and Science University, 3181 Southwest Sam Jackson Park Road, Mail Code: OP32, Portland, OR 97239, USA
E-mail address: dalem@ohsu.edu

Clin Geriatr Med 36 (2020) 131–139
https://doi.org/10.1016/j.cger.2019.09.006
0749-0690/20/Published by Elsevier Inc.

(approximately one-third of patients) sustained fall-related fractures. In a logistic regression analysis of causes of falls, female sex and mean modified Morse Fall Scale score were independently associated with fall-related fractures. The modified Morse Fall Scale is an 85-point scale that accounts for history of falls, secondary diagnoses, need for an ambulatory aid, gait transferring, and mental status, with higher numbers representing worse function. The odds of women sustaining a fall-related fracture were 3.8 times the odds in men. A mean modified Morse Fall score of 72.5 predicted fall-related fractures with 72% sensitivity and 70% specificity. The investigators recommend bone density assessment for all women with PD and for patients with PD with a modified mean Morse Fall score of greater than 72.5.

ORTHOPEDIC INTERVENTIONS FOR SHOULDER PROBLEMS IN PARKINSON DISEASE

Shoulder pain is a common complaint in PD. Shoulder pain caused by rigidity can be a presenting symptom of PD. Patients may seek orthopedic consultation for shoulder pain before receiving a PD diagnosis, and subsequent dopaminergic therapy may relieve their discomfort. Nonetheless, structural musculoskeletal deficits may additionally accompany shoulder rigidity caused by PD. One study found that 22 out of 33 patients with PD had abnormal findings on shoulder ultrasonography, specifically tendon tearing (most commonly the supraspinatus tendon, in 15 out of 22 patients).[3] Longer disease duration contributed to the likelihood of tendon tearing, and increased rigidity was associated with a risk of adhesive capsulitis.

There is a particular risk of anterior-superior shoulder dislocation in PD. Normally anterior-superior displacement of the humerus is rare because the coracoacromial arch prevents superior movement of the humeral head, but in PD the combination of a disrupted supraspinatus tendon and hypertonicity of the deltoid increase the risk of anterior-superior dislocation.[4] Anterior-superior dislocation may even occur after previous shoulder repair, particularly after a fall on the repaired same shoulder.[4]

Several studies have examined complications and outcomes for standard total shoulder arthroplasty (TSA) in PD. Koch and colleagues[5] conducted a retrospective case series of 15 patients with PD at Mayo (Hoehn and Yahr [H&Y] stage II–III) after TSA with a 5-year average follow-up. The surgeries were performed mainly for osteoarthritis; a minority of patients had an underlying diagnosis of osteonecrosis[4] or rheumatoid arthritis.[1] Three out of 15 patients required revision surgery for subluxation caused by a combination of increased shoulder girdle muscle tone and glenoid loosening.[5] Only 25% had excellent or satisfactory functional results on postoperative abduction, external rotation, and internal rotation ratings. The investigators noted that the quality of soft tissues compromises functional results for TSA in patients with PD, especially patients aged 65 years or older. Nonetheless, most patients' pain scores improved significantly after surgery. In a subsequent Mayo study, Kryzak and colleagues[6] assessed a retrospective cohort of 43 shoulder surgeries in patients with PD and osteoarthritis. Patients were followed for a longer period (either 8 years or until the time of any required revision). Eight revisions were required: 3 for early postoperative stability, 4 for loosening hardware, and 1 for perioperative fracture. Factors that predicted fewer overall complications included no preexisting rotator cuff tear, no preoperative moderate or severe subluxation, and the presence of adequate support for postoperative care. About 50% of patients reported unsatisfactory functional results. The risk of an unsatisfactory result was not related to age, sex, or H&Y score.

More recently investigators have explored complications and functional outcomes of other methods of surgical interventions for shoulder instability beyond TSA. TSA is the standard surgical intervention that uses an anterior approach. Other methods include hemiarthroplasty (HA) and reverse shoulder arthroplasty (RSA). In HA, the humeral head is replaced with a prosthesis and the glenoid (socket) is left intact. In RSA, surgeons take a reverse approach for the joint arthroplasty.

In a retrospective review, Kryzak and colleagues[7] examined 7 hemiarthroplasties in patients with PD (primarily H&Y stage III, mean age 72 years). After an average 10 years of follow-up, 3 out of 7 patients still reported moderate to severe pain or limited function. Postoperative complications included poor union of the greater tuberosity in 4 out of 7 patients and glenohumeral subluxation in 4 out of 7 patients. The investigators thus considered the benefit of HA to be marginal for patients with PD.

Other investigators have additionally focused on short-term perioperative complications of HA and RSA in patients with PD. In 2015, Burrus and colleagues[8] compared a large retrospective cohort of 800 RSA surgeries, 2800 HA surgeries, and 3300 TSA surgeries in patients with PD and in healthy age-matched controls. For all 3 types of surgery, rates of infection, dislocation, revision arthroplasty, and systemic complications were all higher in patients with PD compared with healthy controls. TSA and HA surgeries resulted in more component loosening. Long-term complications and functional outcomes were not assessed in this study.

Functional outcomes of RSA in 10 patients with PD were followed in a careful matched cohort study.[9] To determine whether RSA provides similar functional outcomes in patients with PD compared with healthy controls, subjects were matched based on age, sex, preoperative diagnosis, and length of follow-up. The average age of patients was 76 years and the average length of follow-up was 43 months. Outcome measures included range of motion, Simple Shoulder Test score, American Shoulder and Elbow Society score, visual analog scale for pain, and complication rates. Patients with PD achieved a similar reduction of pain but less improvement in functional outcome after RSA, less consistent improvement in range of motion, and higher complication rates compared with matched controls.

A note on shoulder pain after deep brain stimulation deep brain stimulation (DBS) in PD: inflammation can occur in the glenohumeral joint months after impulse generator (IPG) implantation in the case of preexisting calcific tendinopathy.[10] Lefaucheur and colleagues[10] reported 2 cases of edema buildup around the IPG with associated subacromial bursitis or partial rupture of the supraspinatus muscle (3 weeks and 9 months after IPG implantation, respectively). The proposed mechanism of action is that fibrosis in surrounding neck muscles related to the presence of extension cables causes a muscular imbalance that triggers inflammation, particularly if tendinopathy is already present. The investigators note that IPG pocket inflammation and pain after DBS with associated tendinopathy may be relieved by nonsteroidal antiinflammatory drugs.

Summary

Patients with PD are at particular risk for anterior-superior dislocation of the shoulder related to supraspinatus tendon tearing and shoulder girdle muscle rigidity. A reasonable goal of shoulder surgery in PD is pain reduction rather than a return of range of motion of clinical function.

SPINE SURGERY IN PARKINSON DISEASE

Chronic low back pain and impaired lumbar range of motion are common in patients with PD. A cross-sectional study of 48 patients with PD with chronic low back pain and 50 age-matched controls showed that patients with PD had increased thoracic kyphosis and decreased lumbar lordosis compared with controls.[11] The patients underwent thoracolumbar radiographs, lumbar range of motion tests, neurologic examination, and quality-of-life questionnaires. The patients with PD showed less anterior pelvic tilt, and this imbalance correlated with H&Y scores.

Lumbar deformities and medical complications related to the diagnosis of PD may increase complications of lumbar spinal surgeries in the PD population. A cross-sectional analysis of complications from decompression or decompression and lumbar fusion using the National Inpatient Sample (NIS) was performed through the US Agency for Healthcare Research and Quality from 2001 to 2012.[12] The NIS is the largest all-payer database of US hospital admissions, composed of a stratified sample of 20% of hospitalizations in 1000 hospitals annually. In this analysis, subjects were propensity score matched for age, sex, and race to compare complications in patients with and without PD after lumbar surgeries of 4 levels or less. Posthemorrhagic anemia and red blood cell transfusion were risks in the PD population compared with controls (odds ratio [OR], 1.53 and 1.83, respectively, for decompression alone and OR 4.78 and 2.86, respectively, in decompression and fusion). A different study using the NIS and propensity score matching compared complications after lumbar fusions in PD and non-PD groups and stratified patients by fusion length of 1 to 2 versus 3 or more levels.[13] Longer fusions were associated with more complications in both patients with PD and controls. After fusions of 3 or more levels, the PD group had a greater risk of posthemorrhagic anemia (OR 2.0 in the PD group and 1.7 in the control group) and red blood cell transfusion (OR 3.2 in the PD group and 2.2 in the control group). Neither study accounted for PD severity.

Shah and colleagues[14] recently reported equal complication rates for patients with PD compared with controls following thoracolumbar fusions, although this report also found that longer fusions still present a greater risk of complications. In this retrospective study, 288 patients with PD (mean age, 69.7 years) and 288 controls with at least 2 years of follow-up from New York's Statewide Planning and Research Cooperative system were analyzed. Patients were matched by age, Charlson comorbidity score, and number of fused levels. Patients with PD incurred higher total charges across spinal surgery–related visits ($187,807 vs $126,610; $P<.001$), but rates of medical complications (35.8% PD vs 34.0% no PD; $P = .662$) and revision surgery (12.2% vs 10.8%; $P>.05$) were comparable. Postoperative mortalities were comparable between PD and non-PD cohorts (2.8% vs 1.4%; $P = .243$). Logistic regression identified 9-level or higher spinal fusion as a significant predictor for an increase in total complications (OR, 5.64) for patients with PD and controls; PD was not associated with increased odds of any adverse outcomes. This recent report suggests that patients with PD who undergo thoracolumbar fusions incur higher hospital charges compared with patients without PD, but have comparable complication and revision rates.

McClelland and colleagues[15] used the NIS to retrospectively assess the socioeconomic impact of lumbar fusions of 2 or more levels in patients with PD and in matched control subjects. Length of stay more than 1 week, total hospital charges greater than $200,000, and nonroutine discharge disposition were all significantly increased in the PD group. The study was not powered to comment on the role of fusion length, and PD severity was again not assessed.

An increased risk of postoperative delirium after spinal surgeries has been reported in patients with PD. In a large retrospective matched-pair cohort study of 1423 patients with PD and 5498 matched controls in Japan's nationwide inpatient database, PD was a significant predictor of major postoperative complications after all spinal surgeries, even after adjusting for risk factors such as demographics, preoperative comorbidities, duration of anesthesia, and need for blood transfusion during surgery.[16] Postoperative delirium occurred in 30.3% of patients with PD and 5.1% of controls (almost 7-fold higher in patients with PD). This study may have overestimated the risk of postoperative delirium by not capturing the mildest (untreated) patients with PD, because patients with PD were identified by the presence of dopaminergic therapies in their medical records. A case-control study of lumbar decompressions without fusions in 36 patients with PD with a mean H&Y of 2.2, 72 control subjects, and an average follow-up of 1.3 years did not replicate the prior study's results of high postoperative delirium in the PD group, although length of stay, urinary tract infections, and falls were more common in the PD group postoperatively.[17]

Postoperative delirium risk may be higher after spinal surgeries when patients have preexisting hyposmia and rapid eye movement (REM) behavior disorder. In a prospective study of 104 patients not yet diagnosed with PD,[18] hyposmia and REM behavior disorder were significant independent risk factors for postoperative delirium after elective spinal surgery (insomnia, depression, anxiety, constipation, and orthostatic hypotension were not).

Functional results of large lumbar fusions in patients with PD are guarded. In a multicenter retrospective cohort of fusions of 5 levels or more in patients with PD (48 patients, 7 centers, average patient age 67 years, average follow-up of 27 months), 42% of patients required surgical revision.[19] In this study, 42% of patients underwent surgery for low back pain and the remainder for functional impairment. One-third of patients had good results on functional and radiographic assessment, one-third had doubtful results, and one-third of surgeries were determined to be failures. The likelihood of a good result increased with better baseline clinical spinal balance in the standing position. Spinal imbalance is the degree to which spinal impairment affects gait. Unified Parkinson Disease Rating Scale and H&Y scores were not assessed in this study.

A preliminary study showed that interventions for isolated lumbar disc herniations in patients with PD are more successful. Fifteen patients with PD underwent 1-level transforaminal percutaneous endoscopic discectomy (TPED) at L3 to L4, L4 to L5, or L5 to S1.[20] In TPED procedures, surgeons access the intervertebral foramen and the anatomic triangle of Kambin under fluoroscopic guidance with the patient positioned in the lateral decubitus position. Only anesthesia and mild sedation are required, and patients are commonly discharged within 24 hours. Pain (Oswestry Disability Index) and quality of life (Short Form 36) scales were recorded 1 year after surgery. Both pain and disability remained improved. Data on severity of PD or comorbidities were not collected.

Less information is available regarding outcomes of cervical spinal surgery. Xiao and colleagues[21] performed a retrospective matched cohort study of 21 patients with PD with cervical myelopathy compared with 21 control patients with cervical myelopathy. The patients with PD had an average PD history of 5 years. The average extent of the surgical intervention was 4 spinal levels and most surgeries performed were laminectomy and fusion or anterior cervical discectomy and fusion. Cervical pain in patients with PD improved, but overall the patients with PD showed less improvement on the Nurick myelopathy scale. Worse motor outcomes in the PD cohort were mainly noted in the lower extremities. The investigators reported motor and sensory outcomes in the upper extremities in patients with PD that were comparable with those of controls. This study was limited by lack of baseline data regarding cervical curvature and duration of myelopathy symptoms.[22]

Summary

Patients with PD have an increased thoracic kyphosis, decreased lumbar lordosis, and decreased anterior pelvic tilt compared with patients without PD. Lumbar deformities and medical complications related to the diagnosis of PD may increase the complications of lumbar spinal surgeries in PD, particularly in the case of longer fusions. Hyposmia and REM behavior disorder may increase the risk of postoperative delirium after spinal surgeries.

KNEE AND HIP SURGERY IN PARKINSON DISEASE

Imbalances in the hip and knee joint can significantly impair postural stability in patients with PD. Knee extensor (quadriceps) strength, in particular, is often diminished. Nocera and colleagues[23] conducted a cross-sectional study of 44 patients with PD (mean H&Y, 2.3; mean age, 66 years) to investigate the relationship between knee extensor strength and dynamic postural stability when transitioning postures. The investigators measured knee extensor strength with a dynamometer and calculated dynamic postural stability using the center of pressure (COP)–center of mass (COM) moment arm. The COP-COM moment arm is the ability of an individual to tolerate a separation of their COP and COM. This study showed that a lower COP-COM moment arm when transitioning postures (or impaired dynamic postural stability) correlates with impaired knee extensor strength in patients with Parkinson disease. The investigators thus suggest that a program of knee extensor strengthening may be helpful in PD. This study did account for the presence or absence of freezing, festination, dyskinesia, or dystonia.

Recommendations for total knee arthroplasty (TKA) in patients with PD follow from the concern for impaired knee extension in the PD population. More constrained prosthetic devices are recommended for increased stability and decreased risk of anterior tibial displacement, particularly in the case of severe flexion deformity/extensor deficit rigidity. These devices include cruciate-retaining, condylar-constrained kinetic or hinged devices.[24] Regional anesthesia is recommended to minimize the complications of general anesthesia, and sciatic blockade is preferred to isolated femoral blockade to reduce the risk of postoperative flexion contracture.[24] TKA should be avoided in cases of preoperative flexion contracture greater than 25° or lack of response to diagnostic bupivacaine hydrochloride injection (to confirm osteoarthritis pain vs pain caused by PD rigidity).

A recent large study by Newman and colleagues[25] evaluated short-term perioperative complications of TKA in more than 31,000 patients with PD using the NIS. Patients with PD were propensity score matched in a 1:3 ratio with more than 95,000 heathy controls based on age, sex, ethnicity, Charlson Comorbidity Index, and insurance type. The odds of perioperative complications in the PD group were 44 times the odds of perioperative complication in the control group. The most common complications were postoperative delirium, altered mental status, pneumonia, urinary tract infection, sepsis, and transfusions. Length of stay was 6.5% higher and total hospital charges were 3% higher in the PD group.

Other studies have assessed longer-term complications after knee and hip replacements (TKA and total hip arthroplasty [THA]) in patients with PD. A Finnish nationwide registry-based case-control study compared 857 hip and knee surgeries in PD with an average disease duration of 5 years with 2571 matched controls with 1:3 propensity matching and a mean follow-up of 6 years.[26] Although there was no difference in infection rates, revision rates, or 1-year mortality, patients in the PD group had an increased mean length of stay (21 days vs 13 days) and an increased risk of hip dislocation in the first postoperative year (hazard ratio, 2.33). Only one-third patients in the PD group survived to 10 years. Rondon and colleagues[27] conducted a retrospective review of 52 hips and 71 knees undergoing total joint arthroplasty in PD compared with a control cohort matched on age, body mass index, and comorbidities. In an average follow-up 5 years, approximately 24% of patients with PD required revision surgeries. TKA most commonly required revision for infection and THA for periprosthetic fracture and dislocation.

Although complications of TKA are widely reported in PD, 2 recent studies of functional outcomes of TKA are favorable. Wong and colleagues[28] found no significant differences in range of motion or Oxford Knee Score (a patient-reported questionnaire) in a retrospective cohort of 43 patients with PD and 50 age-matched and sex-matched controls with a 1-year follow-up. Another retrospective cohort study of 13 patients with PD and 13 controls found no significant differences in mean Knee Society Score values or mean range-of-motion values after TKA over a follow-up period ranging from 13 to 44 months.[29] Both studies were limited by a lack of assessment of PD severity and the absence of comorbidity matching.

Summary

Complications of TKA in PD are widely reported but can be reduced by the use of constrained prosthetic devices to increase stability at the knee joint, especially in cases with preexisting flexion contracture. Despite widely reported complications, 2 recent studies of functional outcomes of TKA in patients with PD are favorable.

COGNITIVE DECLINE AND ORTHOPEDIC SURGERIES IN PATIENTS WITH PARKINSON

Cognitive decline also limits the success of orthopedic procedures in patients with PD. A large Taiwanese retrospective cohort study using the National Health Insurance Research Database examined 1-year mortalities after surgery for hip fracture in 6626 elderly patients with dementia, Parkinson disease, or both.[30] After adjusting for demographic, clinical, treatment, and provider factors, Cox regression showed similar 1-year mortalities in patients with dementia and patients with both dementia and Parkinson disease (15.53% and 15.82%, respectively). Patients with Parkinson disease but no dementia had a 1-year mortality of 11.59%, a statistically insignificant difference from control subjects who did not have a neurologic illness (9.22%).

A small, prospective, 1-year longitudinal pilot study from the University of Florida focused on the risk of postoperative cognitive decline in patients with PD undergoing orthopedic spine, knee, or hip surgeries.[31] The study was underpowered, but did show that 80% of patients with PD performed significantly worse than their baseline with regard to processing speed (digit symbol coding) and inhibitory function (Stroop Color and Word Test). This decline from baseline was not observed in control subjects without PD. The investigators hypothesized that postoperative declines in processing speed and inhibitory function in patients with PD may be caused by a combination of alterations in small vessel vascular supply to subcortical nuclei, venous emboli, or neurochemical changes associated with anesthesia.

SUMMARY

Orthopedic complaints are common in patients with PD, but may be undertreated. Fall-related fractures are common in PD, especially in women and in patients with an increased modified Morse Fall score. Patients with PD are at particular risk for anterior-superior dislocation of the shoulder related to supraspinatus tendon tearing and shoulder girdle muscle rigidity. A reasonable goal of shoulder surgery in PD is pain reduction rather than a return of range of motion of clinical function. The chance of complications from lumbar spinal surgeries in patients with PD increases with fusion length. Hyposmia and REM behavior disorder may increase the risk of postoperative delirium after spinal surgeries. Complications of TKA in PD are widely reported but can be reduced by the use of constrained prosthetic devices to increase stability at the knee joint, especially in cases with preexisting flexion contracture. Two recent studies of TKA in patients with PD have shown favorable functional outcomes. Postoperative declines in processing speed and inhibitory function in patients with PD may be seen following orthopedic interventions.

REFERENCES

1. Kim YE, Lee W, Yun JY, et al. Musculoskeletal problems in Parkinson's disease: neglected issues. Parkinsonism Relat Disord 2013;19(7):666–9.
2. Cheng K-Y, Lin W-C, Chang W-N, et al. Factors associated with fall-related fractures in Parkinson's disease. Parkinsonism Relat Disord 2014;20(1):88–92.
3. Koh S-B, Roh J-H, Kim JH, et al. Ultrasonographic findings of shoulder disorders in patients with Parkinson's disease. Mov Disord 2008;23(12):1772–6.
4. Matsuzaki T, Kokubu T, Nagura I, et al. Anterosuperior dislocation of the shoulder joint in an older patient with Parkinson's disease. Kobe J Med Sci 2009;54(5): E237–40.
5. Koch LD, Cofield RH, Ahlskog JE. Total shoulder arthroplasty in patients with Parkinson's disease. J Shoulder Elbow Surg 1997;6(1):24–8.
6. Kryzak TJ, Sperling JW, Schleck CD, et al. Total shoulder arthroplasty in patients with Parkinson's disease. J Shoulder Elbow Surg 2009;18(1):96–9.
7. Kryzak TJ, Sperling JW, Schleck CD, et al. Hemiarthroplasty for proximal humerus fractures in patients with Parkinson's disease. Clin Orthop Relat Res 2010;468(7): 1817–21.
8. Burrus MT, Werner BC, Cancienne JM, et al. Shoulder arthroplasty in patients with Parkinson's disease is associated with increased complications. J Shoulder Elbow Surg 2015;24(12):1881–7.
9. Cusick MC, Otto RJ, Clark RE, et al. Outcome of reverse shoulder arthroplasty for patients with Parkinson's disease: a matched cohort study. Orthopedics 2017; 40(4):e675–80.
10. Lefaucheur R, Maltête D, Bouwyn JP, et al. Shoulder tendinopathy causing inflammation surrounding pulse generator after DBS. Parkinsonism Relat Disord 2014; 20(11):1304–6.
11. Watanabe K, Hirano T, Katsumi K, et al. Characteristics of spinopelvic alignment in Parkinson's disease: comparison with adult spinal deformity. J Orthop Sci 2017;22(1):16–21.
12. Baker JF, McClelland S, Line BG, et al. In-hospital complications and resource utilization following lumbar spine surgery in patients with Parkinson disease: evaluation of the national inpatient sample database. World Neurosurg 2017;106: 470–6.
13. McClelland S, Baker JF, Smith JS, et al. Complications and operative spine fusion construct length in Parkinson's disease: a nationwide population-based analysis. J Clin Neurosci 2017;43:220–3.
14. Shah NV, Beyer GA, Solow M, et al. Spinal fusion in Parkinson's disease patients: a propensity score-matched analysis with minimum 2-year surveillance. Spine 2019;44(14):e846–51.
15. McClelland S, Baker JF, Smith JS, et al. Impact of Parkinson's disease on perioperative complications and hospital cost in multilevel spine fusion: a population-based analysis. J Clin Neurosci 2017;35:88–91.

16. Oichi T, Chikuda H, Ohya J, et al. Mortality and morbidity after spinal surgery in patients with Parkinson's disease: a retrospective matched-pair cohort study. Spine J 2017;17(4):531–7.
17. Westermann L, Eysel P, Hantscher J, et al. The influence of Parkinson disease on lumbar decompression surgery: a retrospective case control study. World Neurosurg 2017;108:513–8.
18. Kim KH, Kang SY, Shin DA, et al. Parkinson's disease-related non-motor features as risk factors for post-operative delirium in spinal surgery. PLoS One 2018;13(4): e0195749.
19. Bouyer B, Scemama C, Roussouly P, et al. Evolution and complications after surgery for spine deformation in patients with Parkinson's disease. Orthop Traumatol Surg Res 2017;103(4):517–22.
20. Kapetanakis S, Giovannopoulou E, Thomaidis T, et al. Transforaminal percutaneous endoscopic discectomy in Parkinson disease: preliminary results and short review of the literature. Korean J Spine 2016;13(3):144.
21. Xiao R, Miller JA, Lubelski D, et al. Clinical outcomes following surgical management of coexisting Parkinson disease and cervical spondylotic myelopathy. Neurosurgery 2017;81(2):350–6.
22. Zhong H, Zhou Z, Liu J, et al. Letter: clinical outcomes following surgical management of coexisting Parkinson disease and cervical spondylotic myelopathy. Neurosurgery 2018;82(2):E65–6.
23. Nocera JR, Buckley T, Waddell D, et al. Knee extensor strength, dynamic stability, and functional ambulation: are they related in Parkinson's disease? Arch Phys Med Rehabil 2010;91(4):589–95.
24. Macaulay W, Geller JA, Brown AR, et al. Total knee arthroplasty and Parkinson disease: enhancing outcomes and avoiding complications. J Am Acad Orthop Surg 2010;18(11):687–94.
25. Newman JM, Sodhi N, Wilhelm AB, et al. Parkinson's disease increases the risk of perioperative complications after total knee arthroplasty: a nationwide database study. Knee Surg Sports Traumatol Arthrosc 2019;27(7):2189–95.
26. Jämsen E, Puolakka T, Peltola M, et al. Surgical outcomes of primary hip and knee replacements in patients with Parkinson's disease: a nationwide registry-based case-controlled study. Bone Joint J 2014;96-B(4):486–91.
27. Rondon AJ, Tan TL, Schlitt PK, et al. Total joint arthroplasty in patients with Parkinson's disease: survivorship, outcomes, and reasons for failure. J Arthroplasty 2018;33(4):1028–32.
28. Wong EH, Oh LJ, Parker DA. Outcomes of primary total knee arthroplasty in patients with Parkinson's disease. J Arthroplasty 2018;33(6):1745–8.
29. Ergin ÖN, Karademir G, Şahin K, et al. Functional outcomes of total knee arthroplasty in patients with Parkinson's disease: a case control study. J Orthop Sci 2019. https://doi.org/10.1016/j.jos.2019.06.003 [pii:S0949-2658(19)30184-8].
30. Chiu H-C, Chen C-M, Su T-Y, et al. Dementia predicted one-year mortality for patients with first hip fracture: a population-based study. Bone Joint J 2018; 100-B(9):1220–6.
31. Price CC, Levy S-A, Tanner J, et al. Orthopedic surgery and post-operative cognitive decline in idiopathic Parkinson's disease: considerations from a pilot study. J Parkinsons Dis 2015;5(4):893–905.

Driving in Parkinson Disease

Maud Ranchet, PhD[a], Hannes Devos, PhD[b], Ergun Y. Uc, MD[c,d,*]

KEYWORDS

- Parkinson disease • Driving • Cognition • Transport

KEY POINTS

- Driving is impaired in most patients with Parkinson disease (PD) because of motor, cognitive, and visual dysfunction.
- Driving impairments in PD may increase risk of crashes and result in early driving cessation with loss of independence.
- Drivers with PD should undergo comprehensive evaluations to determine fitness to drive with periodic follow-up evaluations as needed.
- Research in rehabilitation of driving and automation to maintain independence of patients with PD is in progress.

Parkinson disease (PD) impairs driving because of motor, cognitive, and visual dysfunction. The aim of this review is to summarize the evidence on current driving assessment and rehabilitation practices for drivers with PD.

EPIDEMIOLOGY OF DRIVING ISSUES IN PARKINSON DISEASE

The crash risk in PD is not well established.[1] A large survey from Germany indicated that 15% of drivers with PD were involved in car crashes within the last 5 years.[2] Despite reports of increased crash risk, especially in advanced stages of PD,[3] epidemiologic studies on older drivers[4,5] and a recent meta-analysis[6] showed that PD was not associated with higher risk of crashes, consistent with a prospective cohort

Disclosure Statement: Dr. Uc received the following grants: R01 NS044930, NINDS; Merit Review Award 1 I01RX000170, Rehabilitation R&D Branch, US Department of Veterans Affairs. Other authors have nothing to disclose.
[a] Laboratoire Ergonomie Sciences Cognitives pour les Transports (LESCOT), IFSTTAR (Institut Français des Sciences et Technologies des Transports, de l'Aménagement et des Réseaux), 25, Avenue François Mitterrand, Case 24, Cité des Mobilités, Lyon, Bron F-69675, France; [b] Department of Physical Therapy and Rehabilitation Science, Kansas University, KU Medical Center, 3901 Rainbow Boulevard/MS2002, Kansas City, KS 66160, USA; [c] Department of Neurology, University of Iowa, University of Iowa Hospitals and Clinics, 200 Hawkins Drive, Iowa City, IA 52242, USA; [d] Neurology Service, Veterans Affairs Medical Center, 601 Highway 6 W, Iowa City, IA 52246, USA
* Corresponding author. Department of Neurology, University of Iowa, University of Iowa Hospitals and Clinics, 200 Hawkins Drive, Iowa City, IA 52242.
E-mail address: ergun-uc@uiowa.edu

study.[7] Possible explanations include self-regulation using compensatory strategies (eg, avoiding difficult situations) or early driving cessation.[7]

NEUROLOGICAL SUBSTRATES OF DRIVING ISSUES

Studies on brain activation patterns during driving simulation using functional MRI or PET revealed a network of active brain regions associated with vision, perception, visuomotor integration, motor control, and executive functions. Different regions were activated based on the task and driving circumstances. Alcohol or distraction led to disturbances in the activations patterns of these networks that correlated with impairments of driving performance.[8]

PD pathologic condition involves many regions in the brain, leading to multiple cognitive, visual, and motor impairments that can interfere with driving performance at different levels. For example, decreased decision-making ability/executive dysfunction because of frontostriatal dysfunction can lead to poor strategic and tactical choices, such as driving under challenging conditions and making risky maneuvers. Impairments in attention, visual perception, memory, executive functions, motor speed, and self-monitoring can lead to driver errors at the operational level with difficulty in maintaining lane position and keeping a safe distance from other vehicles, and reacting to sudden hazards.[8]

NATURALISTIC STUDIES

Naturalistic studies are complementary to on-road and simulator studies. This approach examines the driving habits and behaviors of drivers in normal and critical situations. Self-regulation practices may also be observed. To date, only 1 naturalistic study has been conducted in drivers with PD to examine whether they show more restrictive patterns than age- and gender-matched controls.[9] Participants were driving in their own vehicle. For 2 weeks, information regarding their driving was recorded with electronic devices, such as distance traveled, duration, and speed. Patients restricted their driving practices to a greater extent than controls. They drove significantly less overall, closer to home, less at night, and less on days with bad weather. They adjusted their travel route by avoiding high-speed roads.[9]

SIMULATOR STUDIES

Driving simulators assess driving behavior in a controlled and reproducible environment. Patients with PD had increased reaction time, greater inaccuracy of steering, slower speed of movement,[10,11] and more collisions than age-matched controls.[12] Drivers with PD had poorer vehicle control compared with controls under normal lighting conditions, but their ability deteriorated much further in low visibility settings (fog), and they had slower reactions and more collisions in response to an illegally incurring vehicle at an intersection.[13] They approached traffic signals at a slower speed, with delayed deceleration,[14] which suggests that they drove more cautiously than controls. They traveled slower around curves, with difficulties maintaining lane positions and difficulties stopping in time.[14–16] The presence of a concurrent task while driving a simulator negatively impacted driving behavior of both healthy older individuals and patients.[15] Tests of updating information in working memory and mental flexibility while driving a simulator showed specific impairments of executive functions in PD.[17] In the updating task, patients with PD recalled fewer road signs than controls while driving, suggesting an updating impairment in mild to moderate stages of PD. These results on the driving simulator were consistent with those obtained from the neuropsychological tests. Repeat testing of the same cohort 2 years after the initial assessment showed that patients with PD had a significantly greater decline in cognitive flexibility than controls.[18] Furthermore, significant decline in flexibility was associated with deterioration in their driving. Driving simulators may also be useful to predict fitness to drive decisions in patients with PD. In addition to a screening battery, scores on the driving simulator helped to better discriminate drivers who passed or failed a formal driving evaluation.[19]

ROAD STUDIES

Drivers with PD committed more driving errors on a standardized on-road driving test compared with control drivers, leading to higher fail rates.[20] The fail rate of drivers with PD ranged between 30% and 56%, whereas the fail rate of control drivers ranged between 0% and 24%.[21–28] Compared with controls, drivers with PD experienced more problems, including the use of signals,[29,30] pedals,[30] and steering wheel.[29,30] As a result, drivers with PD had more difficulties maintaining lane.[21,31,32] Drivers with PD also showed more difficulties adapting their speed to the traffic flow[27,29,32] and drove slower than controls.[33] These difficulties with speed adaptation particularly emerged when driving while distracted.[34] The most important driving performance predictors of failure in the road test were difficulties in turning left at intersections, lane maintenance at low speed, and speed adaptations at high speed.[35] Clinical predictors of failure were older age, higher motor impairment, postural instability/gait disorder subtype, and impaired visual acuity, scanning, information processing speed and attention,[35] and executive dysfunction, especially impaired updating and mental flexibility.[27]

Furthermore, drivers with PD anticipated and responded less accurately to road signs,[21,30,31] traffic lights,[30] other road users,[21] and potentially dangerous road situations.[21]

Drivers with PD also exhibited difficulties navigating intersections,[21,29,32] particularly at T-junctions.[29,30] They also made more errors making left turns[24,25,31] and right turns against traffic.[24]

Drivers with PD had more difficulties negotiating roundabouts,[27] maintaining headway distance,[27] merging into traffic,[24,25] and changing lanes.[24,31,32] They checked their mirrors and blind spots less frequently[21,29,32] and identified less road signs and landmarks along a strip.[34] In addition, drivers with PD were more likely to get lost in traffic while driving a memorized route.[33] A longitudinal cohort study showed that driving safety of patients with PD declined significantly more steeply compared with controls, although the patients who returned for repeat testing 2 years later had a similar performance to controls at baseline and had performed better than the drivers with PD who did not return for repeat testing.[36]

DRIVING REHABILITATION

Driving rehabilitation strategies include training underlying abilities (eg, motor function, information processing speed, or executive functions) or focusing on driving skills. Research on training underlying abilities with driving as an outcome measure in PD is limited. However, driving simulator training has been investigated as a tool to retrain driving and related cognitive skills in several pilot studies in PD. The focus of simulator-based training programs is to expose drivers to different driving situations in dynamic and realistic conditions, aiming to improve the impaired driving skills, or lead to strategies that compensate for impaired driving skills.[37] The simulator training program follows the same principles of motor learning, in which a task-specific driving activity is trained repetitively and intensively. These driving scenarios can be tailored to the needs of the drivers and increase in difficulty to continue challenging the drivers throughout the training sessions. Immediate feedback can be provided through video replay functions so that the drivers can actively participate in identifying their challenges and provide solutions to overcome these challenges.[37] A potential issue of simulator training is the simulator adaptation syndrome (similar to motion sickness) because of mismatch between the simulator's visual cues of movement and the subject's kinesthetic and vestibular cues of being stationary.[37]

In the first pilot study,[38] drivers with PD completed training sessions in a driving simulator that mimicked multiple intersections of varying visibility and traffic load where an incurring vehicle posed a crash risk. After training, participants had fewer crashes and responded faster to the incurring vehicle. However, it is impossible to ascertain at this stage whether these improvements are the result of an actual training effect or rather familiarity with the simulated environment and scenarios. In a follow-up study by the same group, 4 drivers with PD who performed poorly on an on-road driving test completed sessions using the same scenarios reported before[38] as well as various scenarios on decision making, hazard perception, and response behavior. All participants improved their performance on the simulator tasks after training. In addition, most participants completed the on-road driving test with fewer errors.[39] In another pilot study, drivers with PD completed 10 hours of simulator training, individually customized according to their pretraining performance on specific on-road driving skills.[40] After training, participants performed better on a general test of cognitive functions and a test of visual scanning. Moreover, clinically relevant improvements in on-road driving were observed on individual level. The individuals who passed the road test before training passed at posttraining as well. A few individuals who did not pass at pretraining were cleared to drive after training.[40]

POLICY ISSUES

There are currently no uniform legal criteria to guide individuals with PD and health care professionals on fitness to drive. A consensus statement by an Expert Panel Group involving the National Highway Traffic Administration and the American Occupational Therapy Association[41] provided general recommendations on fitness-to-drive decision making according to PD disease severity. Individuals with low motor severity and no/few risk factors (eg, age >75) are usually deemed fit to drive. A comprehensive baseline driving evaluation is recommended to establish baseline fitness to drive with annual follow-up driving evaluations. Retirement from driving is recommended for patients in an advanced motor stage and multiple risk factors. This advice should be conveyed to the driver, and reporting to the driving license agencies should be considered according to the local jurisdiction. Continued consultation on transportation alternatives should be provided to patient and caregiver. For the at-risk group, that is, those individuals with moderate symptoms of PD, comprehensive driving evaluations and planning for driving retirement should be continued. Research is still ongoing to identify the best predictors that determine fitness to drive. Each patient should be evaluated individually using a comprehensive battery testing motor function, cognition, vision, and incorporating other nonmotor aspects, such as sleep, mood, and autonomic dysfunction.

FUTURE OF DRIVING IN PARKINSON DISEASE

With the population aging, the advances in autonomous vehicle technology offer promise for maintaining or improving safe transportation, mobility, and quality of life. The International Society of Automotive Engineers[42] and the National Highway

Safety Administration[43] define 6 levels of driving automation, ranging from no driving automation (level 0) to full driving automation (level 6). In all levels of automation other than full automation, the driver will need to drive the vehicle at least under some conditions. In the level 1, the vehicle has a single aspect of automation that assists the driver with Adaptive Driver Assistance Systems (ADAS). In level 2, the vehicle is able to automate certain parts of the driving experience with more than 1 ADAS aspect. The effect of ADAS on intersection behavior, speed, and headway control was compared in 9 drivers with PD and 9 controls. Both groups showed more confidence using ADAS after several training sessions. Drivers with PD had longer minimum time to collision (TTC) to crossing traffic and crossed less often with a critical TTC to oncoming traffic than older drivers.[44] In the speed and headway control experiment, the speedometer changed color when drivers exceeded the speed limit by more than 10% or 15%. Headway warnings showed up on the screen when drivers were following too close to the lead vehicle. Although ADAS improved outcomes in both groups, removing ADAS after short-term exposure led to deterioration of performance in all speed measures in the PD group.[45] To date, few studies in older adults investigated highest level of automation, such as the level 3, whereby the participant needs to take control of the vehicle.[46–49] Future research should include different age groups of older drivers, including those with PD, to investigate both their opinions regarding vehicle automation and their behavior during the transition phase between manual driving and automated driving.

SUMMARY

Driving is impaired in most patients with PD and progressively worsens resulting in early driving cessation and possibly increased risk of crashes. Although general guidelines on fitness to drive have been proposed, each patient should be evaluated individually with periodic follow-up. Research on rehabilitation of driving skills in PD and automation of driving to maintain vehicular mobility is in progress.

REFERENCES

1. Homann CN, Suppan K, Homann B, et al. Driving in Parkinson's disease–a health hazard? J Neurol 2003;250(12):1439–46.
2. Meindorfner C, Körner Y, Möller JC, et al. Driving in Parkinson's disease: mobility, accidents, and sudden onset of sleep at the wheel. Mov Disord 2005;20(7): 832–42.
3. Dubinsky RM, Gray C, Husted D, et al. Driving in Parkinson's disease. Neurology 1991;41(4):517–20.
4. Hu PS, Trumble DA, Foley DJ, et al. Crash risks of older drivers: a panel data analysis. Accid Anal Prev 1998;30(5):569–81.
5. Lafont S, Laumon B, Helmer C, et al. Driving cessation and self-reported car crashes in older drivers: the impact of cognitive impairment and dementia in a population-based study. J Geriatr Psychiatry Neurol 2008;21(3):171–82.
6. Thompson T, Poulter D, Miles C, et al. Driving impairment and crash risk in Parkinson disease: a systematic review and meta-analysis. Neurology 2018;91(10): e906–16.
7. Uc EY, Rizzo M, Johnson AM, et al. Real-life driving outcomes in Parkinson disease. Neurology 2011;76(22):1894–902.

8. Uc EY. Driving in Parkinson's disease. In: Pfeiffer RF, Ebadi M, Wszolek ZK, editors. Parkinson's disease. 2nd edition. Boca Raton (FL): Taylor & Francis; 2013. p. 1221–44.

9. Crizzle AM, Myers AM. Examination of naturalistic driving practices in drivers with Parkinson's disease compared to age and gender-matched controls. Accid Anal Prev 2013;50:724–31.

10. Lings S, Dupont E. Driving with Parkinson's disease. A controlled laboratory investigation. Acta Neurol Scand 1992;86(1):33–9.

11. Madeley P, Hulley JL, Wildgust H, et al. Parkinson's disease and driving ability. J Neurol Neurosurg Psychiatry 1990;53(7):580–2.

12. Zesiewicz TA, Cimino CR, Malek AR, et al. Driving safety in Parkinson's disease. Neurology 2002;59(11):1787–8.

13. Uc EY, Rizzo M, Anderson SW, et al. Driving under low-contrast visibility conditions in Parkinson disease. Neurology 2009;73(14):1103–10.

14. Stolwyk RJ, Charlton JL, Triggs TJ, et al. Neuropsychological function and driving ability in people with Parkinson's disease. J Clin Exp Neuropsychol 2006;28(6):898–913.

15. Stolwyk RJ, Triggs TJ, Charlton JL, et al. Effect of a concurrent task on driving performance in people with Parkinson's disease. Mov Disord 2006;21(12):2096–100.

16. Stolwyk RJ, Triggs TJ, Charlton JL, et al. Impact of internal versus external cueing on driving performance in people with Parkinson's disease. Mov Disord 2005;20(7):846–57.

17. Ranchet M, Paire-Ficout L, Marin-Lamellet C, et al. Impaired updating ability in drivers with Parkinson's disease. J Neurol Neurosurg Psychiatr 2011;82(2):218–23.

18. Ranchet M, Broussolle E, Paire-Ficout L. Longitudinal executive changes in drivers with Parkinson's disease: study using neuropsychological and driving simulator tasks. Eur Neurol 2016;76(3–4):143–50.

19. Devos H, Vandenberghe W, Nieuwboer A, et al. Predictors of fitness to drive in people with Parkinson disease. Neurology 2007;69(14):1434–41.

20. Devos H, Ranchet M, Emmanuel Akinwuntan A, et al. Establishing an evidence-base framework for driving rehabilitation in Parkinson's disease: a systematic review of on-road driving studies. NeuroRehabilitation 2015;37(1):35–52.

21. Classen S, Brumback B, Monahan M, et al. Driving errors in Parkinson's disease: moving closer to predicting on-road outcomes. Am J Occup Ther 2014;68(1):77–85.

22. Classen S, McCarthy DP, Shechtman O, et al. Useful field of view as a reliable screening measure of driving performance in people with Parkinson's disease: results of a pilot study. Traffic Inj Prev 2009;10(6):593–8.

23. Classen S, Witter DP, Lanford DN, et al. Usefulness of screening tools for predicting driving performance in people with Parkinson's disease. Am J Occup Ther 2011;65(5):579–88.

24. Grace J, Amick MM, D'Abreu A, et al. Neuropsychological deficits associated with driving performance in Parkinson's and Alzheimer's disease. J Int Neuropsychol Soc 2005;11(6):766–75.

25. Heikkilä VM, Turkka J, Korpelainen J, et al. Decreased driving ability in people with Parkinson's disease. J Neurol Neurosurg Psychiatry 1998;64(3):325–30.

26. McCarthy MP, Garvin C, Lanford DN, et al. Clinical predictors of on-road driving performance in patients with Parkinson's disease. Mov Disord 2007;22(Suppl 16):S175.

27. Ranchet M, Paire-Ficout L, Uc EY, et al. Impact of specific executive functions on driving performance in people with Parkinson's disease. Mov Disord 2013;28(14): 1941–8.
28. Worringham CJ, Wood JM, Kerr GK, et al. Predictors of driving assessment outcome in Parkinson's disease. Mov Disord 2006;21(2):230–5.
29. Cordell R, Lee HC, Granger A, et al. Driving assessment in Parkinson's disease–a novel predictor of performance? Mov Disord 2008;23(9):1217–22.
30. Lee H, Falkmer T, Rosenwax L, et al. Validity of driving simulator in assessing drivers with Parkinson's disease. Adv Transport Stud 2007;S81–90.
31. Uc EY, Rizzo M, Johnson AM, et al. Road safety in drivers with Parkinson disease. Neurology 2009;73(24):2112–9.
32. Wood JM. Quantitative assessment of driving performance in Parkinson's disease. J Neurol Neurosurg Psychiatry 2005;76(2):176–80.
33. Uc EY, Rizzo M, Anderson SW, et al. Impaired navigation in drivers with Parkinson's disease. Brain 2007;130(9):2433–40.
34. Uc EY, Rizzo M, Anderson SW, et al. Driving with distraction in Parkinson disease. Neurology 2006;67(10):1774–80.
35. Devos H, Vandenberghe W, Tant M, et al. Driving and off-road impairments underlying failure on road testing in Parkinson's disease. Mov Disord 2013;28(14): 1949–56.
36. Uc EY, Rizzo M, O'Shea AMJ, et al. Longitudinal decline of driving safety in Parkinson disease. Neurology 2017;89(19):1951–8.
37. Akinwuntan AE, Devos H. Driving rehabilitation. In: Wilson R, Raghavan P, editors. Stroke rehabilitation. St Louis (MO): Elsevier; 2018. p. 225–33.
38. Dawson JD, Rizzo M, Anderson SW, et al. Collision avoidance training using a driving simulator in drivers with Parkinson's disease: a pilot study. Proc Int Driv Symp Hum Factors Driv Assess Train Veh Des 2009;2009:154–60.
39. Uc E, Rizzo M, Anderson S, et al. Driver rehabilitation in Parkinson's disease using a driving simulator: a pilot study. Proc Int Driv Symp Hum Factors Driv Assess Train Veh Des 2011;2011:248–54.
40. Devos H, Morgan JC, Onyeamaechi A, et al. Use of a driving simulator to improve on-road driving performance and cognition in persons with Parkinson's disease: a pilot study. Aust Occup Ther J 2016;63(6):408–14.
41. Classen S, National Highway Traffic Safety Administration, American Occupational Therapy Association. Consensus statements on driving in people with Parkinson's disease. Occup Ther Health Care 2014;28(2):140–7.
42. Society of Automotive Engineers International (SAE). Taxonomy and definitions for terms related to driving automation systems for on-road motor vehicles. Warendale (PA: SAE International; 2016. Report No.: 2016-09-30. Available at: https:// www.sae.org/content/j3016_201609. Accessed April 12, 2019.
43. National Highway Traffic Safety Administration (NHTSA). The road to full automation. Washington, DC: NHTSA; 2018. Available at: https://www.nhtsa.gov/ technology-innovation/automated- vehicles-safety. Accessed April 12, 2019.
44. Dotzauer M, Caljouw SR, de Waard D, et al. Intersection assistance: a safe solution for older drivers? Accid Anal Prev 2013;59:522–8.
45. Dotzauer M, Caljouw SR, De Waard D, et al. Longer-term effects of ADAS use on speed and headway control in drivers diagnosed with Parkinson's disease. Traffic Inj Prev 2015;16(1):10–6.
46. Clark H, Feng J. Age differences in the takeover of vehicle control and engagement in non-driving-related activities in simulated driving with conditional automation. Accid Anal Prev 2017;106:468–79.

47. Körber M, Gold C, Lechner D, et al. The influence of age on the take-over of vehicle control in highly automated driving. Transp Res Pt F-traffic Psychol Behav 2016;39: 19–32.

48. Miller D, Johns M, Ive HP, et al. Exploring transitional automation with new and old drivers. Warrendale (PA): SAE International; 2016. Report No.: 2016-01–1442. Available at: https://www.sae.org/publications/technical-papers/content/2016-01-1442/. Accessed April 12, 2019.

49. Molnar LJ, Ryan LH, Pradhan AK, et al. Understanding trust and acceptance of automated vehicles: an exploratory simulator study of transfer of control between automated and manual driving. Transp Res Pt F-traffic Psychol Behav 2018;58: 319–28.

Palliative Care for Parkinson Disease

Hillary D. Lum, MD, PhD[a,b], Benzi M. Kluger, MS, MD[c,*]

KEYWORDS

- Parkinson disease • Palliative care • Caregiver • Goals of care
- Advance care planning

KEY POINTS

- Palliative care (PC) aims to relieve suffering for persons affected by serious illness by addressing medical, psychosocial, and spiritual needs.
- Parkinson disease (PD) causes distress related to medical, emotional, social, and spiritual needs beginning at the time of diagnosis and throughout the entire course of the disease.
- PC approaches may improve quality of life for individuals with PD and their families throughout the course of the illness.
- A primary PC approach to PD includes providing the diagnosis and prognosis with compassion, discussing goals of care and advance care planning, systematic assessment of motor and nonmotor symptoms including psychosocial issues, and timely hospice referrals.

RELEVANCE OF PALLIATIVE CARE TO PARKINSON DISEASE

The World Health Organization defines palliative care (PC) as "an approach that improves the quality of life of patients and families facing life-threatening illness, through the prevention and relief of suffering by means of early identification and impeccable assessment and treatment of pain and other problems, physical, psychosocial and spiritual."[1] Advances in PC relevant to Parkinson disease (PD) include the following: (1) recognition that PC needs may emerge at any point of an illness, including at the time of initial diagnosis; (2) PC may be effectively delivered in diverse settings including outpatient clinics; (3) PC may be integrated into standard disease-focused therapies; and (4) PC may be delivered by clinicians not specializing in PC, so-called primary PC.[2,3]

Disclosure: The authors have nothing to disclose.
[a] Division of Geriatric Medicine, Department of Medicine, University of Colorado Denver, University of Colorado Anschutz Medical Campus, Mail Stop C-293, 12631 East 17th Avenue, Aurora, CO 80045, USA; [b] Eastern Colorado VA Geriatric Research Education and Clinical Center, Aurora, CO, USA; [c] Department of Neurology, University of Colorado Denver, University of Colorado Anschutz Medical Campus, Mail Stop B-185, 12631 East 17th Avenue, Aurora, CO 80045, USA
* Corresponding author.
E-mail address: benzi.kluger@ucdenver.edu

Clin Geriatr Med 36 (2020) 149–157
https://doi.org/10.1016/j.cger.2019.09.013
0749-0690/20/© 2019 Elsevier Inc. All rights reserved.

geriatric.theclinics.com

Despite significant morbidity and mortality (the Centers for Disease Control lists PD as the 14th leading cause of death[4]), there are many areas where persons living with PD have unmet PC needs under current models of care. Patients report that receiving the diagnosis of PD is traumatic and frequently given without acknowledging psychosocial consequences.[5] Nonmotor symptoms such as pain and depression are undertreated, and other psychosocial issues such as caregiver support are rarely addressed.[6,7] Most patients with PD do not receive hospice care and most of then die in hospitals or other institutions.[8,9]

Growing evidence suggests that PC needs contribute to quality of life (QOL) in PD and that PC approaches may improve both QOL and symptom burden and reduce hospital deaths.[10–13] There are a growing number of centers now offering PC for PD.[14] In this article, the authors focus on primary PC skills relevant to PD, including providing a diagnosis and prognosis with compassion; discussing goals of care; complex symptom management; caregiver support; addressing social, emotional, and spiritual well-being; and discussing hospice (**Box 1**).

Providing Diagnosis and Prognosis with Compassion

There are few events as significant to patients as receiving their PD diagnosis.[15] Although physicians may choose to focus on the relatively positive aspects of this diagnosis, namely that medical and other therapies can significantly improve many symptoms, they should not underestimate the potential impact of this diagnosis on patients and their families. Physicians can improve the experience by responding empathetically to emotional reactions, sharing information, and listening to the patient's hopes and expectations. Clinicians should provide adequate time for these conversations and anticipate a need for close follow-up to prevent feelings of confusion and abandonment. Consider these communication approaches:

- SPIKES mnemonic for important conversations: *S*etting up the Interview; *A*ssessing patient's *P*erception; Obtaining patient's *I*nvitation; Giving *K*nowledge; Addressing *E*motions; Strategy and *S*ummary.[16]
  - Within this mnemonic the authors highlight a few points. When getting an *I*nvitation, be prepared for patients and their caregivers to have different desires for how much information they want. For *K*nowledge, it is important to let patients know how the diagnosis is made but not to overwhelm them. For the *S*ummary step, the authors recommend having an opportunity for follow-up

---

Box 1
Primary palliative care skills for neurodegenerative illnesses

- Providing a diagnosis and prognosis with compassion
- Discussing goals of care
  - Assessing decision-making capacity
  - Advance care planning and advance directives
  - Anticipatory guidance for future needs
- Complex symptom management
- Caregiver support
- Addressing social, emotional, and spiritual well-being
- Referring to hospice care

within a few weeks, as patients and families may need time to process this information and may not hear everything that is said at the first visit.

- NURSE mnemonic to address emotions: *N*ame the emotion; *U*nderstand and legitimize the emotion; *R*espect the challenges and courage of the patient; *S*upport the patient and family; *E*xplore approaches to working with this emotion.[17]
- Prognosis discussions: consider questions of "How long?" and "How well?" when addressing prognosis, while tailoring the conversation to individual preferences.[18]

Discussing Goals of Care

In goals of care discussions, patients, families, and clinicians work together to develop guidelines for current and future care.[19] Patients and family members share their values, hopes, and fears, and clinicians provide information regarding diagnosis, prognosis, and guidance on medical treatments and resources. Important issues to address include what activities are most important to maintain QOL and how the patient and family would like to navigate ongoing or increasing levels of patient dependence. The following questions are helpful in order to better understand patients' and families' values: How do you define QOL? What do you enjoy or look forward to? What is the toughest part of this? What are you most afraid of?

1. Assessing Decision-Making Capacity: goals of care conversations should be initiated early due to the possibility of progressive cognitive impairment. Clinicians should be careful not to overemphasize the primacy of patient desires when they lack capacity, nor to discount the desires of patients with the capacity to provide input despite mild to moderate dementia.[20] Capacity is best assessed in relation to specific decisions rather than globally and can be assessed by remembering 4 "C"s (a patient's ability to understand their Condition, their Choices, the Consequences of choices, and Consistency of decisions over time).
2. Advance Care Planning (ACP) and Advance Directives: ACP is a process that includes identifying a legal health care surrogate decision maker, discussing personal values, documenting preferences in an advance directive, and translating preferences into medical care plans.[21] Recognizing the importance of ACP as part of high-quality PD care, the American Academy of Neurology Parkinson Disease Quality Measurement Set recommends annual review of advance directives and designated health care surrogates.[22,23] One approach to discussing ACP is to ask about advance directives and health care surrogates as part of your social history; this helps normalize the conversation and signals that it is a routine part of good care. It may also be prudent to not delve deeply into ACP when first giving the diagnosis to avoid overwhelming the patient. Evidence-based, state-specific advance directives designed to have low cognitive burden are available (https://prepareforyourcare.org/advance-directive).[24] The advance directives should be easily accessible and shared with the health care surrogate, other family members, and health care providers. A patient's ability to engage in ACP in PD may be influenced by specific perceptions and misperceptions of ACP and symptoms (eg, apathy, cognitive dysfunction).[25] Optimal engagement of patients with PD and caregivers should proactively address misperceptions of ACP and use interdisciplinary team members (ie, social workers, nurses, others) to incorporate ACP into routine PD care.
3. Anticipatory Guidance for Future Needs: in addition to decision-making related to ACP, many individuals with PD will face difficult life transitions. A PC approach can incorporate open and ongoing conversations about decisions related to the

medical impact on employment, living situation, financial, and safety concerns. One of the medical team's primary responsibilities is to screen for safety concerns. The presence of safety issues may mandate the clinician to modify or even challenge previously stated goals of care and to play the "bad guy" in advocating for decisions that go against the patient's wishes (eg, memory care placement) to avoid blame among family members.

Individuals with PD have increased risk of motor vehicle accidents.[26] Although state laws vary, the authors recommend patients with red flags (eg, family or patient brings up driving concerns, significant vision, motor or cognitive impairment) to either stop driving or get a specialty driving evaluation. Firearms and other potentially dangerous items should be secured, particularly from patients with psychotic symptoms. Verbal, physical, or sexual threats or abuse may be directed at either the caregiver or patient and may be more common in PD than previously believed.[27] Financial risk may arise through scams targeting persons with impaired cognition or through spending by patients with poor judgment.[28] Falls and wandering may necessitate 24/7 supervision or placement in patients with advanced disease or dementia, and wearable identification, fall alert systems, and home safety evaluations are recommended to try to preclude placement.[29]

Complex Symptom Management

Patient QOL in PD is heavily driven by nonmotor issues and these symptoms are underrecognized by clinicians.[6] As a part of routine care, the authors recommend systematic assessment of pain, mood, psychotic and behavioral symptoms, sleep and energy, communication, autonomic symptoms, swallowing, and nutrition.[30]

Pain is a common symptom in PD and a focused history and examination may reveal causes of pain that are related to PD and can respond to targeted treatments (eg, nocturnal leg cramps, off dystonia).[31] Unfortunately, even with appropriate therapies, many sources of pain may not be eliminated and can become chronic sources of suffering. A PC approach to this chronic pain includes understanding the physical aspects of the pain, as well as its functional, psychological, and social impact. Clinicians should talk with patients about their goals for pain management, emphasizing that functional improvement may be more attainable than complete pain elimination and that side effects of medications must be weighed against function. A proactive approach should be taken to avoid preventable pain (eg, keeping joints mobilized, good skin care in bed- or chair-bound individuals) and treatment should be directed at specific causes when possible. Opioids may be used judiciously in PD, with a recommendation to start with short-acting opioids and keeping a focus on function if possible (eg, using an acetaminophen-hydrocodone tablet a few times a week before physical therapy or other life-affirming activities).[32]

Sleep disorders and fatigue are common and may affect both patient and caregiver well-being. Management requires identifying and treating contributing factors such as depression, specific sleep disturbances, anemia, pain, and medications, particularly dopamine agonists that can contribute to excessive daytime sleepiness and even daytime sleep attacks.[33] Nonpharmacologic approaches include exercise, energy conservation strategies, mindfulness training, cognitive behavioral therapy, or acupuncture.[33,34]

PD can lead to dysphagia, weight loss, and changes in appetite. These symptoms may be important prognostic indicators and can be used to support hospice referrals.[35] Modifications to diet should be made within the context of an individual's goals of care. For example, patients may forego pureed diets and choose to continue eating their favorite foods if they place a higher value on the pleasures of eating than minimizing risk of aspiration. Feeding tubes are rarely indicated in these conditions, and evidence does not support their use to prevent aspiration or prolong survival.[36] Enteral feeding may be considered when prolonged and difficult mealtimes reduce QOL, when dysphagia is advanced out of proportion to other signs of disease progression, or if maintaining artificial nutrition is consistent with goals of care.

Caregiver Support

Individuals with PD often develop long-term disabilities and rely on family members to meet daily care needs. Unfortunately, family caregivers frequently suffer from sleeplessness, fatigue, anxiety, depression, guilt, and impaired immunologic responses. Caregiver burden is defined by perceptions of adverse consequences of caregiving to emotional, social, financial, physical, and spiritual functioning.[37] Risk factors for caregiver burden include female sex, low education, residing with the care recipient, depression, social isolation, financial stress, higher number of caregiving hours, and lack of choice in caregiver role.[38] Distressed caregivers often develop negative attitudes toward the disease and relationship problems with the patient and other family and experience complex bereavement.[39]

Attending to the health and well-being of family caregivers may be facilitated through interdisciplinary clinics including social work and counseling resources.[40] The National Consensus Development Conference for Caregiver Assessment recommends the following approach: (1) identify primary and additional caregivers; (2) incorporate needs and preferences of both the patient and caregiver in all care planning; (3) improve caregivers' understandings of their roles and teach them the skills necessary to carry out the tasks of caregiving; and (4) recognize the need for periodic reassessment of care outcomes for the patient and caregiver.[38]

Clinicians can also perform a brief assessment of caregiver well-being or use a formal assessment tool.[41] In addition to detecting caregiver issues early and making appropriate referrals, even brief inquiries directed to caregivers are deeply appreciated and let the caregiver know they are not alone.[42]

Protective factors against caregiver burden include resilience, perceived competence, self-efficacy, social support, optimism, and emphasis on the positive aspects of care.[39] Some of these protective characteristics can be trained through targeted interventions. Available support for caregivers include educational materials, home health care or skilled nursing support, respite care, advocacy organizations, and local or online support groups.

Addressing Social, Emotional, and Spiritual Well-Being

PC goes beyond the medical model of psychiatric illness to embrace the many social, emotional, and spiritual issues that arise during serious illness. PD challenges personhood in numerous ways including independence, social relationships, sense of identity, and appearance.[43] Social activity is critical for maintaining cognitive ability and social isolation adversely affects QOL and mortality in PD.[44] Social activity can be promoted through awareness, community organizations, and social work.

It is important to distinguish common but difficult emotional reactions to chronic illness from the psychiatric syndromes of anxiety and depression and to provide encouragement and support to patients and families who may already experience shame around these feelings. Common difficult emotions include grief, guilt, frustration, demoralization, anger, and fears about the future including financial issues, death, or dementia.[5,7,42,43,45] These emotions are frequently driven by spiritual or existential issues including hopelessness, meaninglessness, loneliness, and death anxiety.[46] The search for meaning is one of the central coping mechanisms when facing progressive illness and may buffer against depression, hopelessness, and desire for hastened death among terminally ill patients. Spirituality and religion also may provide meaning, and these factors may guide patient decision-making during illness. Chaplains or other spiritual guides may provide emotional and spiritual support, particularly for patients adverse to the idea of psychotherapy.[47] Other interventions that enhance meaning and build resilience include traditional psychotherapy, mindfulness-based approaches, gratitude journals, and narrative-based approaches.[48,49]

Referring to Hospice

Hospice refers to PC at the end of life. In the United States, the Medicare hospice benefit is available to patients certified by 2 physicians to have a prognosis of 6 months or less. Hospice is fully covered for Medicare, Veterans Affairs beneficiaries, and most Medicaid and private insurances. The authors recommend 3 questions to facilitate hospice discussions and referrals. First, would the patient and family benefit from the services available from hospice? Hospice is commonly delivered in the home or current residence and includes education, caregiver support, and a team of visiting nurses, social workers, chaplains, volunteers, and bereavement support for the family. Second, are the patient's and family's goals of care aligned with hospice? A helpful question is, "If you were to develop a serious pneumonia, would you want to go to a hospital for intravenous fluids and antibiotics?" If the answer is no and the goals of care are comfort, hospice may be appropriate. If the answer is yes, one may consider home PC or other home services. Finally, does the patient qualify for hospice? Although there are limited empirical data[35] and no formal guidelines specific to PD, the authors advocate a proactive approach to referring appropriate patients to hospice by documenting the following: accelerating rate of progression, weight loss, dysphagia, falls, hospitalizations, and withdrawal from activities. One may also use Medicare Hospice Guidelines for "Dementia," "Adult Failure to Thrive," or "Neurologic Illness" if they apply, recognizing that these guidelines often lead to late referrals if strictly followed.

SUMMARY

PC issues are common in PD and a PC approach may improve the QOL of patients and family caregivers. Primary PC can be integrated into PD care and management through ongoing discussions about goals of care, assessment and management of a broad range of physical, emotional, social, and spiritual needs, attending to caregivers, and appropriate referrals to hospice.

REFERENCES

1. WorldHealthOrganization. WHO definition of palliative care [online]. 2016. Available at:http://www.who.int/cancer/palliative/definition/en/. . Accessed August 28, 2016.
2. Strand JJ, Kamdar MM, Carey EC. Top 10 things palliative care clinicians wished everyone knew about palliative care. MayoClin Proc 2013;88(8):859–65.
3. Quill TE, Abernethy AP. Generalist plus specialist palliative care–creating a more sustainable model. N Engl J Med 2013;368(13):1173–5.
4. Murphy S, Kochanek K. Deaths: preliminary data for 2010. Natl Vital Stat Rep 2012;60:1–52.

5. Hall K, Sumrall M, Thelen G, et al, 2015 Parkinson's Disease Foundation sponsored "Palliative Care and Parkinson's Disease" Patient Advisory Council. Palliative care for Parkinson's disease: suggestions from a council of patient and carepartners. NPJParkinsons Dis 2017;3(1):16.

6. Shulman LM, Taback RL, Rabinstein AA, et al. Non-recognition of depression and other non-motor symptoms in Parkinson's disease. ParkinsonismRelatDisord 2002;8(3):193–7.

7. Goy ER, Carter JH, Ganzini L. Needs and experiences of caregivers for family members dying with Parkinson disease. J PalliatCare 2008;24(2):69–75.

8. Moens K, Houttekier D, Van den Block L, et al. Place of death of people living with Parkinson's disease: a population-level study in 11 countries. BMCPalliatCare 2015;14:28.

9. Snell K, Pennington S, Lee M, et al. The place of death in Parkinson's disease. Age Ageing 2009;38(5):617–9.

10. Kluger BM, Shattuck J, Berk J, et al. Definingpalliative care needs in Parkinson's disease. MovDisordClinPract 2019;6(2):125–31.

11. Miyasaki JM, Long J, Mancini D, et al. Palliative care for advanced Parkinson disease: an interdisciplinary clinic and new scale, the ESAS-PD. Parkinsonism RelatDisord 2012;18(Suppl3):S6–9.

12. Tuck KK, Zive DM, Schmidt TA, et al. Life-sustaining treatment orders, location of death and co-morbid conditions in decedents with Parkinson's disease. ParkinsonismRelatDisord 2015;21(10):1205–9.

13. Veronese S, Gallo G, Valle A, et al. Specialist palliative care improves the quality of life in advanced neurodegenerative disorders: NE-PAL, a pilot randomised controlled study. BMJ Support Palliat Care 2017;7(2):164–72.

14. Kluger BM, Fox S, Timmons S, et al. Palliative care and Parkinson's disease: meeting summary and recommendations for clinical research. ParkinsonismRelatDisord 2017;37:19–26.

15. Phillips LJ. Dropping the bomb: the experience of being diagnosed with Parkinson's disease. GeriatrNurs 2006;27(6):362–9.

16. Baile WF, Buckman R, Lenzi R, et al. SPIKES-A six-step protocol for delivering bad news: application to the patient with cancer. Oncologist 2000;5(4):302–11.

17. VitalTalk.Responding to emotion. 2018. Available at:https://www.vitaltalk.org/guides/responding-to-emotion-respecting/. . Accessed April 20, 2019.

18. Holloway RG, Gramling R, Kelly AG. Estimating and communicating prognosis in advanced neurologic disease. Neurology 2013;80(8):764–72.

19. Sinuff T, Dodek P, You JJ, et al. Improving end-of-life communication and decision making: the development of a conceptual framework and quality indicators. J PainSymptomManage 2015;49(6):1070–80.

20. Abu Snineh M, Camicioli R, Miyasaki JM. Decisional capacity for advanced care directives in Parkinson's disease with cognitive concerns. ParkinsonismRelatDisord 2017;39:77–9.

21. Sudore RL, Lum HD, You JJ, et al. Definingadvance care planning for adults: a consensus definition from a multidisciplinary delphipanel. J PainSymptomManage 2017;53(5):821–32.e1.

22. Factor SA, Bennett A, Hohler AD, et al. Quality improvement in neurology: Parkinson disease update quality measurement set: executive summary. Neurology 2016;86(24):2278–83.

23. Petrillo LA, McMahan RD, Tang V, et al. Older adult and surrogate perspectives on serious, difficult, and important medical decisions. J Am Geriatr Soc 2018;66(8):1515–23.

24. Sudore RL, Schillinger D, Katen MT, et al. Engaging diverse English- and Spanish-speaking older adults in advance care planning: the PREPARE randomized clinical trial. JAMA Intern Med 2018;178(12):1616–25.

25. Lum HD, Jordan SR, Brungardt A, et al. Framingadvance care planning in Parkinson's disease: patient and care partner perspectives. Neurology 2019;92: e2571–9.

26. Uc EY, Rizzo M, O'shea AM, et al. Longitudinal decline of driving safety in Parkinson disease. Neurology 2017;89(19):1951–8.

27. Bruno V, Mancini D, Ghoche R, et al. High prevalence of physical and sexual aggression to caregivers in advanced Parkinson's disease. Experience in the palliative care program. ParkinsonismRelatDisord 2016;24:141–2.

28. Verbaan D, van Rooden SM, Visser M, et al. Psychotic and compulsive symptoms in Parkinson's disease. MovDisord 2009;24(5):738–44.

29. Schrag A, Hovris A, Morley D, et al. Caregiver-burden in Parkinson's disease is closely associated with psychiatric symptoms, falls, and disability. ParkinsonismRelatDisord 2006;12(1):35–41.

30. Bernal-Pacheco O, Limotai N, Go CL, et al. Nonmotor manifestations in Parkinson disease. Neurologist 2012;18(1):1–16.

31. Ha AD, Jankovic J. Pain in Parkinson's disease. MovDisord 2012;27(4):485–91.

32. Trenkwalder C, Chaudhuri KR, Martinez-Martin P, et al. Prolonged-release oxycodone-naloxone for treatment of severe pain in patients with Parkinson's disease (PANDA): a double-blind, randomised, placebo-controlled trial. Lancet Neurol 2015;14(12):1161–70.

33. Herlofson K, Kluger BM. Fatigue in Parkinson's disease. J Neurol Sci 2017;374: 38–41.

34. Kluger BM, Rakowski D, Christian M, et al. Randomized, controlled trial of acupuncture for fatigue in Parkinson's disease. MovDisord 2016;31(7):1027–32.

35. Goy ER, Bohlig A, Carter J, et al. Identifying predictors of hospice eligibility in patients with Parkinson disease. Am J HospPalliatCare 2015;32(1):29–33.

36. Stavroulakis T, McDermott CJ. Enteral feeding in neurological disorders. Pract Neurol 2016;16(5):352–61.

37. Zhong M, Evans A, Peppard R, et al. Validity and reliability of the PDCB: a tool for the assessment of caregiver burden in Parkinson's disease. IntPsychogeriatr 2013;25(9):1437–41.

38. Adelman RD, Tmanova LL, Delgado D, et al. Caregiver burden: a clinical review. JAMA 2014;311(10):1052–60.

39. Palacio C, Krikorian A, Limonero JT. The influence of psychological factors on the burden of caregivers of patients with advanced cancer: resiliency and caregiver burden. PalliatSupport Care 2018;16(3):269–77.

40. Collins LG, Swartz K. Caregiver care. Am FamPhysician 2011;83(11):1309–17.

41. Hagell P, Alvariza A, Westergren A, et al. Assessment of burden among family caregivers of people with Parkinson's disease using the zarit burden interview. J PainSymptomManage 2017;53(2):272–8.

42. Boersma I, Jones J, Coughlan C, et al. Palliative care and Parkinson's disease: caregiver perspectives. J Palliat Med 2017;20(9):930–8.

43. Boersma I, Jones J, Carter J, et al. Parkinson disease patients' perspectives on palliative care needs: what are they telling us? NeurolClinPract 2016;6(3):209–19.

44. Forsaa EB, Larsen JP, Wentzel-Larsen T, et al. Predictors and course of health-related quality of life in Parkinson's disease. MovDisord 2008;23(10):1420–7.

45. Hall K. Window of opportunity: living with the reality of Parkinson's and the threat of dementia. Woodland Park, CO: Pygmy Books, LLC; 2014.

46. Anandarajah G, Hight E. Spirituality and medical practice: using the HOPE questions as a practical tool for spiritual assessment. Am FamPhysician 2001; 63(1):81–9.
47. Richardson P. Spirituality, religion and palliative care. Ann Palliat Med 2014;3(3): 150–9.
48. Guerrero-Torrelles M, Monforte-Royo C, Rodríguez-Prat A, et al. Understanding meaning in life interventions in patients with advanced disease: a systematic review and realist synthesis. Palliat Med 2017;31(9):798–813.
49. Chochinov HM, Hack T, Hassard T, et al. Dignity therapy: a novel psychotherapeutic intervention for patients near the end of life. J ClinOncol 2005;23(24): 5520–5.

Multidisciplinary Care to Optimize Functional Mobility in Parkinson Disease

Anouk Tosserams, MD[a,b,*], Nienke M. de Vries, PT, PhD[b],
Bastiaan R. Bloem, MD, PhD[b], Jorik Nonnekes, MD, PhD[a]

KEYWORDS

- Multidisciplinary care • Parkinson disease • Functional mobility • Gait • Balance

KEY POINTS

- Integrating the services of different health care professionals into a multidisciplinary team approach improves the overall management of persons living with Parkinson disease.
- Previous initiatives have shown that a well-organized multidisciplinary collaborative structure has the potential to improve quality of care and health outcomes, while reducing health care costs. However, more work is needed to define which care model is best for which type of health care issue in Parkinson patients.
- Care should be tailored to the individual patient, for example, by using the International Classification of Functioning, Disability, and Health model as a framework.
- Use of health care innovations, such as wearable telemonitoring devices, is likely to facilitate the delivery of multidisciplinary, personalized care for all patients with Parkinson disease in the near future.

Disclosure Statement: Prof B.R. Bloem currently serves as Associate Editor for the *Journal of Parkinson Disease*, serves on the editorial board of *Practical Neurology* and *Digital Biomarkers*, has received honoraria from serving on the scientific advisory board for Abbvie, Biogen, UCB, and Walk with Path, has received fees for speaking at conferences from AbbVie, Zambon, Roche, GE Healthcare, and Bial, and has received research support from The Netherlands Organisation for Scientific Research, the Michael J. Fox Foundation, UCB, Abbvie, the Stichting Parkinson-Fonds, the Hersenstichting Nederland, the Parkinson Foundation, Verily Life Sciences, Horizon 2020, the Topsector Life Sciences and Health, and the Parkinson Vereniging. Dr J. Nonnekes has received research support from ZonMw and the Michael J. Fox Foundation. The other authors have nothing to disclose.
[a] Department of Rehabilitation, Radboud University Medical Centre, Donders Institute for Brain, Cognition and Behaviour, Reinier Postlaan 4, PO Box 9101, Nijmegen 6500 HB, The Netherlands; [b] Department of Neurology, Radboud University Medical Centre, Donders Institute for Brain, Cognition and Behaviour, Reinier Postlaan 4, PO Box 9101, Nijmegen 6500 HB, The Netherlands
* Corresponding author.
E-mail address: Anouk.Tosserams@radboudumc.nl

Clin Geriatr Med 36 (2020) 159–172
https://doi.org/10.1016/j.cger.2019.09.008
0749-0690/20/© 2019 Elsevier Inc. All rights reserved.

INTRODUCTION

Parkinson disease (PD) is a highly complex neurodegenerative disorder, resulting in a wide variety of motor and nonmotor symptoms. These symptoms can have a disabling impact on the functional capabilities and quality of life of affected persons.[1,2] Despite optimal medical management, with levodopa as the current cornerstone of most management programs, many motor and nonmotor symptoms improve only partially. Therefore, complementary nonpharmacologic interventions, such as physiotherapy, occupational therapy, speech language therapy, are needed to provide optimal care. There is increasing evidence that demonstrates the added value for each of these professional disciplines, when this is offered as a monodisciplinary intervention.[3] The evidence is most abundant and persuasive for a range of physiotherapy interventions, but there are now also good clinical trials to support the merits of other allied health interventions. There is also growing support (largely practice based, but to a much lesser extent evidence based) that integrating these different health care professionals into a multidisciplinary care team may improve the overall management of PD.[4,5] Multidisciplinary care is to be distinguished from interdisciplinary care. In a multidisciplinary team, each individual team member approaches the patient from their own perspective. The decisions made by all separate team members may be integrated by a team leader, but this is not a prerequisite. In contrast, interdisciplinary care emerges from multidisciplinary care when health care professionals make group decisions about patient care.[6,7] Here, the authors focus on "multidisciplinary care" in its broadest sense, and use that as the overarching umbrella term in the remainder of this article.

In this review, the authors elaborate on multidisciplinary care for persons living with PD, by using gait and balance impairments as an example of a treatable target that typically necessitates an integrated approach by a range of different and complementary professional disciplines. Gait and balance impairments are hallmarks of PD and are reckoned among the most disabling symptoms.[8] Their management is complex because dopaminergic treatment is only partially effective, particularly when the disease progresses.[9,10] Complementary nonpharmacologic interventions are therefore needed to provide optimal care, ideally via a multidisciplinary approach.[11] Here, the authors first discuss that for optimal multidisciplinary care, a mere assessment of symptoms (eg, retropulsion test to test balance correcting steps, or a turning test to provoke freezing of gait) is insufficient, and that it is essential to also assess the functional consequences of balance and gait impairments, in combination with interacting personal and environmental factors. The outcome of such a broader assessment will subsequently determine the focus and content of the multidisciplinary treatment program. Finally, the authors elaborate on the various models to organize multidisciplinary care, and on the new possibilities to improve care by integration of technological innovations.

ASSESSMENT OF FUNCTIONAL MOBILITY

Gait and balance impairments result in recurrent falls, fall-related injuries, and a secondary fear of falling.[12,13] The impairments in mobility may impose detrimental consequences for participation of affected individuals at home, at work, or within the community. For example, patients may experience a loss of independence or may be unable to continue their work activities as they did before. Hence, gait and balance impairments can have a very negative impact on functional mobility.

To map functional mobility, the International Classification of Functioning, Disability, and Health (ICF) framework can be of help (as was recently outlined by

Bouca-Machado and colleagues).[14] In the ICF framework (**Fig. 1**), 3 levels of human functioning are identified: (a) body functions and structures (including body impairments), (b) limitations in performing activities, and (c) participation restrictions in daily life.[15] Personal and environmental contextual factors are interconnected with these levels of human functioning.

As shown in **Fig. 1**, body impairments that influence functional mobility in PD can be subdivided into motor symptoms, nonmotor symptoms, and general risk factors. Hypokinetic gait is one of the motor symptoms that impacts functional mobility. Gait in PD is phenotypically characterized by a reduced step height and length, reduced gait speed, an asymmetrically reduced arm swing, a narrow base of support, and a stooped posture.[16] Additional characteristic paroxysmal motor symptoms in PD are festination and freezing of gait (the feeling that the feet suddenly become glued to the floor despite the intention to walk).[8] Balance-correcting steps (another motor symptom impacting functional mobility) are typically small, or not present at all.[17] Importantly, nonmotor symptoms influence functional mobility as well. For example, orthostatic hypotension influences the ability to rise from sit to stance, and executive dysfunction may hamper the ability to perform a dual task (eg, talking while walking, or carrying a tray while walking). Anxiety is another important nonmotor symptom, which is increasingly recognized as an important provoking factor for freezing of gait.[18] In addition to these motor and nonmotor symptoms, general risk factors, such as polyneuropathy or visual impairments, impact functional mobility as well. For example, visual impairments (which are common in PD, because of the disease itself, medication, or comorbid ophthalmologic conditions)[19] may well hamper the ability of patients with PD to use visual cueing to shift from an automatic to goal-directed control of walking. Similarly, a marked polyneuropathy may interfere with the subject's ability to benefit from tactile cues delivered to the feet.

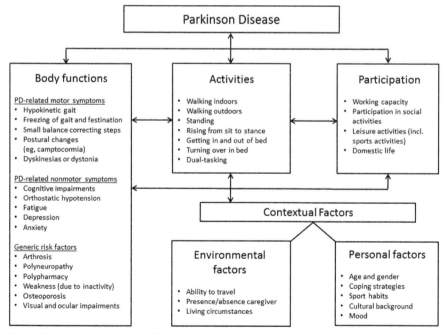

Fig. 1. The ICF framework applied to PD.

These body impairments (because of both motor and nonmotor symptoms as well as general risk factors) influence the activities that a patient is able to perform, and this subsequently impacts their participation in society. For example, the ability to maneuver in crowded places is often difficult for patients because of freezing of gait, and this may hinder their ability to go to a busy marketplace. Another example is the inability to perform a dual task while walking, which may result in an inability to serve coffee to family members.

Assessment of functional mobility is not complete without the evaluation of contextual factors, which can be subdivided into environmental factors and personal factors. The presence or absence of a caregiver aside (eg, proximity to the patient can markedly influence gait), an important environmental factor is represented by the living circumstances. For example, a patient living in an urban area might experience difficulties traveling by subway, whereas a patient living in the countryside may experience difficulties going to the supermarket independently. Knowing that freezing of gait is often provoked by narrow spaces, a home packed with furniture can be detrimental. Personal factors impact functional mobility as well. Coping strategies are an important personal factor: patients may experience difficulties accepting their gait and balance impairments and may feel ashamed to apply cueing strategies that are visible to others. This approach will have a negative impact on their functional mobility. Alternatively, patients may experience difficulties integrating energy-conservation strategies (including an activity-rest balance over the entire day and week) into their daily lives, resulting in an increase of experienced fatigue and a negative impact on functional mobility.

MULTIDISCIPLINARY MANAGEMENT TO IMPROVE FUNCTIONAL MOBILITY

The outcome of the assessment of functional mobility using the ICF framework will determine the focus of the multidisciplinary treatment. Importantly, the focus of the treatment is also largely dependent on the personal aims of the patient. For example, coping strategies may have a negative impact on functional mobility, but when the patient is completely reluctant to improve these, they should not be the focus of the treatment.[20] Focus is also important because patients with PD often experience a lack of energy, and multitarget therapy not tailored to the individual carries a serious risk of hitting nothing.[21] The purpose of this review article is not to describe all possible treatment options in detail, as this has already been done elsewhere.[11,22–24] Instead, the authors elaborate on 1 treatment modality at each level of the ICF framework. As the levels of the ICF framework interact, these treatment modalities will ultimately influence the overall functional mobility of the patient.

Body Functions: Compensation Strategies to Reduce Freezing of Gait

A comprehensive summary of compensation strategies to reduce freezing of gait was recently published.[25] An international group of experts asked patients to videotape self-invented tricks to improve their mobility. From these recording, 59 unique compensation strategies were identified and classified into 7 main categories (**Table 1**). Importantly, the effect of compensation strategies can differ between patients. For example, a particular form of compensation (eg, visual cueing) may have a spectacular effect on gait in 1 patient, but display no effect on, or even worsen, freezing of gait in another.[26,27] Personal preferences may also play a role; some patients do not mind walking around with earbuds that provide rhythmic auditory cueing, whereas others find this socially unacceptable. In that regard, many patients dislike the social stigma that is associated with most visual cueing strategies, because these

Table 1
Classification of compensation strategies for gait impairments in Parkinson disease

Compensation Strategy	Example
1. External cueing	Walking at the rhythm of a metronome
2. Internal cueing	Focusing on predefined components of the gait cycle
3. Changing balance requirements	Weight shifting in place before gait initiation
4. Altering the mental state	Making movements as if being a toreador
5. Action observation/motor imagery	Watching another person walking before gait initiation
6. Adopting a new walking pattern	Walking while lifting the knees high
7. Other forms of using the legs to move forward	Roller skating

Data from Nonnekes J, Ruzicka E, Nieuwboer A, et al. Compensation strategies for gait impairments in Parkinson's disease: a review. JAMA Neurol 2019;76(6):718–25.

are very visible to outsiders. In order to identify the optimal compensation strategies for each patient, patients with PD should be educated about the available compensation strategies and receive guidance from an experienced therapist. At present, this usually turns into an ineffective trial-and-error process. Future studies should therefore evaluate whether there are certain patient characteristics that can predict the most effective compensation strategy in an individual patient. Possible predictive patient characteristics may include the presence of on-state freezing of gait, the specific provoking circumstances for freezing of gait (eg, freezing while turning around in the kitchen may require a different strategy than start akinesia), the presence of cognitive dysfunction, comorbidity, and, as indicated before, personal preferences.[28] Further research is also warranted to obtain a deeper understanding of the underlying working mechanisms of compensation strategies for gait impairments in PD. For example, gait is a complex motor function, but it is largely automated. Patients with PD experience difficulties walking in an automatic manner, because of the loss of dopaminergic innervation in the posterior putamen (a region associated with habitual behavior).[29] Compensation strategies likely enable a shift from automatic to goal-directed gait control. This shift may involve the recruitment of additional cortical areas, and it may be that the nature and extent of these cortical networks differ from patient to patient or from compensation strategy to another. Recent technological advances, such as ambulatory electroencephalography measurements, create opportunities to study the precise involvement of cortical compensatory mechanisms, possibly even at an individual level, thus allowing for more focused delivery of personalized rehabilitation strategies.

Activity Level: Dual-Task Training

An example of an intervention at the activity level is dual-task training. Patients with PD often experience difficulties performing dual tasks while walking.[30,31] Compromised dual-task gait in PD correlates with more freezing of gait, an increase in fall risk, and reduced functional mobility.[32–34] The usefulness of dual-task training in PD has been debated in recent years.[30,35] Controversies also surround the most effective method of dual-task training. In the DUALITY trial,[36] the efficacy of a consecutive versus an integrated approach was assessed as well as the possible fall risk of both training methods. In this multicenter single-blinded study a total of 121 patients with

PD (Hoehn and Yahr stage II–III on medication) were randomized to either the consecutive group in which motor and cognitive tasks were trained separately or the integral group in which motor and cognitive tasks were trained concurrently. After 6 weeks of this at-home training program, led by a physiotherapist, significant improvement in gait velocity during dual-task performance was described in both treatment groups. Both training modes had a similar effect on dual-task gait, and the improvements were preserved at 12-week posttraining follow-up in both groups. In addition, the increase in dual-task gait velocity did not increase the risk of falls in both study arms. These findings suggest that dual-task training is safe and advantageous, and that it should be adopted in clinical practice. According to this trial, there is no particular dual-task training approach that is superior.

Participation Level: Job Coaching

The authors now move to providing an example of an intervention at the participation level. Gait and balance impairments can have a negative impact on the ability to work (eg, a patient with young-onset PD who is unable to continue working as a waiter).[37] Rates of unemployment and early retirement are high in PD and contribute to disease burden. A retrospective study of an Irish cohort of patients with PD, diagnosed before the age of 65 years, found that unemployment rates for men with PD were significantly increased compared with the general Irish population, with a standardized ratio of 1.6. Interestingly, this discrepancy was not present among women. Median retirement age was 58 years for male patients with PD and 61 years for female patients with PD, compared with 63.5 and 65 years, respectively, in the general population.[38] Internal factors that may influence performance and well-being in the workplace in patients with PD involve symptom severity, daily fluctuations in PD symptoms, and coping strategies and adaptability of the patient. An important positive external factor is the presence of supportive, educated employers and colleagues who enable appropriate adjustments to the professional environment.[39] Therefore, job coaching (eg, by an occupational therapist or an occupational doctor) that targets both these internal and external factors should be an element of multidisciplinary care in patients with PD.

Environmental Factors: Adaptations in the Home Setting and Caregiver Strain

A home environment that is not tailored to meet the functional mobility of the patient contributes to falls and is associated with negative health outcomes in PD.[40] Characteristics of the environment can both ameliorate and impede the independence, efficacy, and safety in performing daily activities.[41] Therefore, assessment of the home environment by an occupational therapist, physiotherapist, or Parkinson nurse specialist is essential in patients with gait and balance difficulties. Because persons living with PD generally experience fluctuations in symptoms throughout the day, it is recommended to observe the patient in the home environment during both "on"- and "off" states.[42] Considering this may not be feasible in daily practice, the authors recommend actively inquiring about challenges occurring during the on state or off state at home. Although the necessary adaptations are person and context specific, there is some general advice concerning the home environment. First, creating a free walking and turning route by rearranging furniture and reducing the number of objects present in the room are essential (because freezing often occurs in narrow spaces). Second, potential tripping hazards, such as slippery flooring, doorsteps, loose mats, or electricity cables, should be eliminated. Furthermore, creating support points or seating possibilities during balance-challenging activities, such as getting dressed, should be considered. Because patients with PD with axial symptoms rely more on good vision to compensate for their gait impairments, installing proper lighting solutions (eg, on the route to the toilet at night) should also receive attention. Last, freezers may profit from applying visual cues in places of importance, such as stripes on the floor on the turning route in front of the wardrobe, or a more 3-dimensional approach, such as a painted staircase illusion.[43]

Having to deal with gait and balance impairments of a person with PD may impose significant strain onto the caregiver. Taking on the role of caregiver, in addition to the role of being a partner, family member, or friend, can be challenging.[44] A deterioration of functional mobility can impact caregivers in multiple ways. For example, caregivers often experience stress if their partner or family member with PD falls frequently. Moreover, as a result of their family member's decreased mobility, caregivers may be forced to take on more responsibilities, for example, by taking over certain tasks in the household. These circumstances can markedly affect the caregivers' lives at a physical, emotional, and psychosocial level and, thereby, affect their quality of life. In a postal survey that was conducted among 123 caregivers of persons with PD,[45] more than 40% of caregivers indicated that their health had suffered as a result of caregiving. In addition, almost half of them had increased depression scores, and more than 60% reported that their social life had been negatively affected. Multidisciplinary care should therefore also pay attention to the well-being of the caregiver. Ideally, caregivers are integrated within the multidisciplinary team. The optimal way to organize this collaboration, however, needs to be established. Thus far, most studies on multidisciplinary care models found no effect, or even a negative effect, on experienced caregiver strain.[46,47] In the IMPACT trial,[48] a nonrandomized controlled trial on integrated multidisciplinary care for persons with PD, 301 patients were included from 6 community hospitals in The Netherlands. Patients in the intervention group were offered an individually tailored comprehensive assessment in an expert tertiary referral center followed by dedicated referrals to a regional network of allied health professionals specialized in PD, whereas patients in the control group did not have access to this infrastructure. As a secondary outcome, caregiver strain was assessed using the BELA-A-k at 4 and 8 months. Although the intervention showed no effect on the overall caregiver strain, the results suggested a higher caregiver strain in the intervention group for the partner bonding subscale of the BELA-A-k, perhaps because the well-intended multidisciplinary approach now opened a "Pandora's box" and made caregivers more aware of the vast complexity of PD. Another explanation is the need for the caregiver to now arrange and supervise the many time-consuming visits to members of the multidisciplinary team. Regardless, this paradoxic effect needs to be addressed in future studies.

Personal Factors: Sport Habits

In addition to environmental factors, personal factors, such as sport habits, could also be a target of intervention. An active lifestyle is essential for patients with PD, because there is increasing evidence for a beneficial effect of regular exercise on motor as well as nonmotor functioning.[49,50] Maintaining physical fitness can be challenging for patients with gait and balance impairments, because not all physical activities are feasible or safe for these patients (eg, freezing of gait may lead to falls while playing tennis). Fear of falling especially is a major barrier for physical activity in patients with PD,[51] whereas, on the other hand, fall risk can be reduced by regular physical activity.[52] Many different types of exercise are nowadays available for patients with PD, varying from endurance and strength training to dance, tai chi, and boxing.[3,50] There is accumulating evidence that long-term aerobic-type exercise especially may attenuate PD symptoms[53]; however, recent work also highlights the potential of mind-body exercise, such as mindfulness yoga.[54] Most of these interventions show an overall benefit, even though it remains unclear what frequency, intensity, and duration of exercise are most effective. The issue of dosing was addressed very nicely in the recent SPARX trial,[55] a phase 2 multicenter randomized clinical trial that examined the feasibility and safety of high-intensity treadmill exercise in patients with de novo PD. In total, 128 patients were randomly assigned to 1 of 3 groups: high-intensity exercise (80%–85% of maximum heart rate), moderate-intensity exercise (60%–65% of maximum heart rate), or wait-list control. The intervention groups performed treadmill exercise 4 days per week for 6 months. After 6 months, the high-intensity group, but not the moderate-intensity group, showed a decreased change in Unified Parkinson Disease Rating Scale motor score compared with the control group. Future phase 3 trials are now warranted to determine whether high-intensity exercise is indeed more beneficial compared with moderate-intensity exercise. The European Guideline for Physical Therapy in PD gives an overview of the different exercise options and advices to choose a combination of different types of exercises based on the patient's preference, barriers, and motivators in order to increase long term adherence.[56] Future research needs to focus on the evaluations of the comparative effectiveness of different types of exercise and the long-term benefits.

ORGANIZATION OF MULTIDISCIPLINARY CARE

Because of the wide range of motor and nonmotor problems, a multidisciplinary approach is increasingly being recognized as the best way to manage the disease.[5,57] Multidisciplinary care can take many different forms, but there is no template on how professionals should collaborate optimally. Various models have been tested, with variable success. Although multidisciplinary care is generally accepted to be of great value, the few controlled trials on intramural multidisciplinary care in PD produced inconsistent findings; although some care models established a significant improvement in quality of life and motor performance in patients with PD,[58,59] others showed no effect on the same outcome measures.[48] The heterogeneity of these trials, including research design, nature of multidisciplinary interventions, and methodological strength, further complicates the interpretation of results.[57]

Multidisciplinary care can also be organized in networks that extend beyond the walls of the traditional institutions. The Dutch ParkinsonNet is an example of how this can be organized.[60] ParkinsonNet was founded in 2004 and consists of regional networks that provide specialized care, preferably in the community (close to the patient's home). The core elements of ParkinsonNet include (1) professional empowerment, by educating professionals on PD according on evidence-based guidelines and by concentrating care among these specifically trained professionals through preferred referrals; (2) patient empowerment, by informing patients and including them as partners in health care; and (3) team empowerment, by organizing and supporting care into multidisciplinary, regional networks.[61] These community-based networks can be supported by expert clinics within that region. For example, in the authors' own tertiary center, an expert team of a physiatrist, a physiotherapist, and an occupational therapist is available for consultation regarding gait and balance. Based on this consultation, specific treatment advice can be given to community-based therapists. However, this approach is supported by practice-based evidence only, and clinical studies remain warranted to assess the efficacy and cost-effectiveness of this collaborative structure. Moreover, the feasibility of an international implementation of such an approach will be highly dependent on the different national health care systems.

ParkinsonNet has reached full national coverage in The Netherlands, and currently includes 12 different professional disciplines (eg, physiotherapists, occupational therapists, speech-language therapists, Parkinson nurses) in 70 regional subnetworks.[59] Studies show that ParkinsonNet improves the quality of care, improves health outcomes for patients managed by the network, and reduces health care costs substantially.[61–72] Specifically, a recent analysis of a medical claims database of 4381 patients with PD, spanning an observation period of 3 years, indicated that patients who were treated by a specialized ParkinsonNet physiotherapist experienced fewer PD-related complications (17.3% vs 21.3%) and received fewer physiotherapy treatment sessions (33.7 vs 47.9) as compared with a generically active therapist. Also, specialized physiotherapy was associated with lower annual costs for physiotherapy ($1019 vs $1451) and lower total health care costs ($2245 vs $2824).[72]

The authors expect that other health care innovations can further improve the delivery of optimal multidisciplinary care. One of these innovations includes home-based monitoring as a way to support self-management. Currently, medical decisions are based almost exclusively on periodic in-clinic evaluations. For a variety of reasons, such "snapshots" are unable to capture the actual impact on the patient's functioning in their own home environment. When it comes to functional mobility especially, episodic clinic visits are not well suited to detect relevant changes, such as gradual changes in walking speed or declines in physical activity. Also, it is usually very difficult to obtain a reliable impression of falls and their associated consequences during the brief hospital consultations. Consequently, it is challenging to tailor treatment decisions to the actual needs of patients.

Continuous self-monitoring in the home situation has the potential to markedly improve clinical decision making, by offering feedback to both the patient (by providing them with a tool for self-management and decision support as to when professional support is required) and the clinician (to make better informed treatment decisions).[73] Ideally, self-monitoring uses a combination of wearable sensors for noninvasive and continuous passive ambulatory monitoring[74,75] and longitudinal and repetitive digital self-report.[76,77] An example of such a setup includes the use of body-worn sensors or smartphones that can capture physical activity. The data gathered by the sensors can be linked to a smartphone app (feedback loop) allowing patients to receive feedback on their own activity levels. Importantly, the dashboard in the app may also allow patients to add self-reports on physical activity (ie, type and intensity) and on medication use as well the efficacy of the medication. The latter is essential to gain insight into the development and severity of response-fluctuations, which are typical for PD.[78,79] Such approaches can help to detect whether for any individual patient, freezing and falls predominantly occur when the medication effects have worn off, or when the medication is working well, or when the medication leads to excessive involuntary movements. Moreover, when health professionals would have access to these data, this would give them direct information on patient functioning in daily life, which will allow them to tailor their treatment to the individual patient.

Many studies have demonstrated the technological feasibility of this approach and have shown good (long-term) adherence, both for wearable sensors and for digital self-report.[74,79–82] Telemonitoring is expected to provide relevant insights into the patient's functioning in their own home environment and has the potential to offer a more accurate reflection of the true disability in real daily life. However, many challenges remain to be resolved before this can really be implemented into daily clinical practice.[83] Myriad questions need to be addressed in future studies, such as the optimal number of sensors that a patient should wear, which position (or positions) of the sensor on the body provides the most reliable and useful information, which type of sensor is the most sensitive (eg, smartphone or body worn), as well as a further refinement and validation of data algorithms for the detection of key outcome parameters. Another critical challenge is to study whether the feedback offered by such telemonitoring systems can lead to a sustained behavioral change (ie, improved quality of the decision making) in both patients and professionals.

SUMMARY

Integrating different health care professionals into a multidisciplinary care team is needed to tackle the complexity of PD and, even though the evidence is not consistent and more work is needed, is likely to improve the overall management of PD. Such multidisciplinary care should be tailored to the desires and needs of each individual patient. This personalized form of care can be achieved by assessment of the patient at the level of body function, activity, and participation level, while also considering the context of the patient by focusing on personal and environmental factors. The outcome of this assessment will then determine the focus of the multidisciplinary treatment. Although evidence remains conflicting, several initiatives have shown the potential of a well-organized multidisciplinary collaborative structure to improve quality of care and health outcomes, while reducing health care costs in some examples. With the use of health care innovations, such as wearable telemonitoring devices, the path toward multidisciplinary, personalized care for all patients with PD will continue to develop.

ACKNOWLEDGMENTS

The authors thank C. Scheijmans for her insights concerning the role of the occupational therapist in gait and balance impairment in patients with Parkinson disease.

REFERENCES

1. Global Parkinson's Disease Survey Steering Committee. Factors impacting on quality of life in Parkinson's disease: results from an international survey. Mov Disord 2002;17:60–7.
2. Muslimovic D, Post B, Speelman JD, et al. Determinants of disability and quality of life in mild to moderate Parkinson disease. Neurology 2008;70(23):2241–7.
3. Bloem BR, de Vries NM, Ebersbach G. Nonpharmacological treatments for patients with Parkinson's disease. Mov Disord 2015;30(11):1504–20.
4. Qamar MA, Harington G, Trump S, et al. Multidisciplinary care in Parkinson's disease. Int Rev Neurobiol 2017;132:511–23.
5. Post B, van der Eijk M, Munneke M, et al. Multidisciplinary care for Parkinson's disease: not if, but how! Postgrad Med J 2011;87(1031):575–8.
6. Jessup RL. Interdisciplinary versus multidisciplinary care teams: do we understand the difference? Aust Health Rev 2007;31(3):330–1.
7. Radder DLM, de Vries NM, Riksen NP, et al. Multidisciplinary care for people with Parkinson's disease: the new kids on the block! Expert Rev Neurother 2019;19(2): 145–57.
8. Nutt JG, Bloem BR, Giladi N, et al. Freezing of gait: moving forward on a mysterious clinical phenomenon. Lancet Neurol 2011;10(8):734–44.
9. Schaafsma JD, Balash Y, Gurevich T, et al. Characterization of freezing of gait subtypes and the response of each to levodopa in Parkinson's disease. Eur J Neurol 2003;10(4):391–8.
10. Smulders K, Dale ML, Carlson-Kuhta P, et al. Pharmacological treatment in Parkinson's disease: effects on gait. Parkinsonism Relat Disord 2016;31:3–13.

11. Nonnekes J, Snijders AH, Nutt JG, et al. Freezing of gait: a practical approach to management. Lancet Neurol 2015;14(7):768–78.
12. Bloem BR, Hausdorff JM, Visser JE, et al. Falls and freezing of gait in Parkinson's disease: a review of two interconnected, episodic phenomena. Mov Disord 2004; 19:871–84.
13. Canning CG, Paul SS, Nieuwboer A. Prevention of falls in Parkinson's disease: a review of fall risk factors and the role of physical interventions. Neurodegener Dis Manag 2014;4(3):203–21.
14. Bouca-Machado R, Maetzler W, Ferreira JJ. What is functional mobility applied to Parkinson's disease? J Parkinsons Dis 2018;8(1):121–30.
15. Leonardi M, Meucci P, Ajovalasit D, et al. ICF in neurology: functioning and disability in patients with migraine, myasthenia gravis and Parkinson's disease. Disabil Rehabil 2009;31(Suppl 1):S88–99.
16. Nonnekes J, Goselink RJM, Ruzicka E, et al. Neurological disorders of gait, balance and posture: a sign-based approach. Nat Rev Neurol 2018;14(3):183–9.
17. Nonnekes J, de Kam D, Geurts AC, et al. Unraveling the mechanisms underlying postural instability in Parkinson's disease using dynamic posturography. Expert Rev Neurother 2013;13(12):1303–8.
18. Ehgoetz Martens KA, Shine JM, Walton CC, et al. Evidence for subtypes of freezing of gait in Parkinson's disease. Mov Disord 2018;33(7):1174–8.
19. Ekker MS, Janssen S, Seppi K, et al. Ocular and visual disorders in Parkinson's disease: common but frequently overlooked. Parkinsonism Relat Disord 2017; 40:1–10.
20. Prochaska JO, Norcross JC. Stages of change. Psychother Theor Res Pract Train 2001;38(4):443–8.
21. Nonnekes J, Nieuwboer A. Towards personalized rehabilitation for gait impairments in Parkinson's disease. J Parkinsons Dis 2018;8(s1):S101–6.
22. Maetzler W, Nieuwhof F, Hasmann SE, et al. Emerging therapies for gait disability and balance impairment: promises and pitfalls. Mov Disord 2013;28(11): 1576–86.
23. Alves Da Rocha P, McClelland J, Morris ME. Complementary physical therapies for movement disorders in Parkinson's disease: a systematic review. Eur J Phys Rehabil Med 2015;51(6):693–704.
24. Kim SD, Allen NE, Canning CG, et al. Postural instability in patients with Parkinson's disease. Epidemiology, pathophysiology and management. CNS Drugs 2013;27(2):97–112.
25. Nonnekes J, Ruzicka E, Nieuwboer A, et al. Compensation strategies for gait impairments in Parkinson's disease: a review. JAMA Neurol 2019. https://doi.org/10. 1001/jamaneurol.2019.0033.
26. Stummer C, Dibilio V, Overeem S, et al. The walk-bicycle: a new assistive device for Parkinson's patients with freezing of gait? Parkinsonism Relat Disord 2015; 21(7):755–7.
27. Dietz MA, Goetz CG, Stebbins GT. Evaluation of a modified inverted walking stick as a treatment for parkinsonian freezing episodes. Mov Disord 1990;5:243–7.
28. Nieuwboer A. Cueing for freezing of gait in patients with Parkinson's disease: a rehabilitation perspective. Mov Disord 2008;23(Suppl 2):S475–81.
29. Redgrave P, Rodriguez M, Smith Y, et al. Goal-directed and habitual control in the basal ganglia: implications for Parkinson's disease. Nat Rev Neurosci 2010; 11(11):760–72.

30. Kelly VE, Eusterbrock AJ, Shumway-Cook A. A review of dual-task walking deficits in people with Parkinson's disease: motor and cognitive contributions, mechanisms, and clinical implications. J Parkinsons Dis 2012;2012:918719.

31. Rochester L, Galna B, Lord S, et al. The nature of dual-task interference during gait in incident Parkinson's disease. Neuroscience 2014;265:83-94.

32. Heinzel S, Maechtel M, Hasmann SE, et al. Motor dual-tasking deficits predict falls in Parkinson's disease: a prospective study. Parkinsonism Relat Disord 2016;26:73-7.

33. Spildooren J, Vercruysse S, Desloovere K, et al. Freezing of gait in Parkinson's disease: the impact of dual-tasking and turning. Mov Disord 2010;25(15): 2563-70.

34. Fuller RL, Van Winkle EP, Anderson KE, et al. Dual task performance in Parkinson's disease: a sensitive predictor of impairment and disability. Parkinsonism Relat Disord 2013;19(3):325-8.

35. Strouwen C, Molenaar EA, Münks L, et al. Dual tasking in Parkinson's disease: should we train hazardous behavior? Expert Rev Neurother 2015;15(9): 1031-1039.

36. Strouwen C, Molenaar EALM, Münks L, et al. Training dual tasks together or apart in Parkinson's disease: results from the DUALITY trial. Mov Disord 2017;32(8): 1201-10.

37. Banks P, Lawrence M. The disability discrimination act, a necessary, but not sufficient safeguard for people with progressive conditions in the workplace? The experiences of younger people with Parkinson's disease. Disabil Rehabil 2006; 28(1):13-24.

38. Murphy R, Tubridy N, Kevelighan H, et al. Parkinson's disease: how is employment affected? Ir J Med Sci 2013;182:415-9.

39. Mullin RL, Chaudhuri KR, Andrews TC, et al. A study investigating the experience of working for people with Parkinson's and the factors that influence workplace success. Disabil Rehabil 2018;40(17):2032-9.

40. Jonasson SB, Ullen S, Iwarsson S, et al. Concerns about falling in Parkinson's disease: associations with disabilities and personal and environmental factors. J Parkinsons Dis 2015;5(2):341-9.

41. Kamsma YPT. Implications of motor and cognitive impairments for ADL and motor treatment of patients with Parkinson's disease. Ned Tijdschr Fysioth 2004;114(3): 59-62 [in Dutch].

42. Foongsathaporn C, Panyakaew P, Jitkritsadakul O, et al. What daily activities increase the risk of falling in Parkinson patients? An analysis of the utility of the ABC-16 scale. J Neurol Sci 2016;364:183-7.

43. Janssen S, Soneji M, Nonnekes J, et al. A painted staircase illusion to alleviate freezing of gait in Parkinson's disease. J Neurol 2016;263(8):1661-2.

44. Mosley PE, Moodie R, Dissanayaka N. Caregiver burden in Parkinson disease: a critical review of recent literature. J Geriatr Psychiatry Neurol 2017;30(5):235-52.

45. Schrag A, Hovris A, Morley D, et al. Caregiver-burden in Parkinson's disease is closely associated with psychiatric symptoms, falls, and disability. Parkinsonism Relat Disord 2006;12(1):35-41.

46. Trend P, Kaye J, Gage H, et al. Short-term effectiveness of intensive multidisciplinary rehabilitation for people with Parkinson's disease and their carers. Clin Rehabil 2002;16(7):717-25.

47. Wade DT, Gage H, Owen C, et al. Multidisciplinary rehabilitation for people with Parkinson's disease: a randomised controlled study. J Neurol Neurosurg Psychiatry 2003;74(2):158-62.

48. van der Marck MA, Bloem BR, Borm GF, et al. Effectiveness of multidisciplinary care for Parkinson's disease: a randomized, controlled trial. Mov Disord 2013; 28(5):605–11.

49. Goodwin VA, Richards SH, Taylor RS, et al. The effectiveness of exercise interventions for people with Parkinson's disease: a systematic review and meta-analysis. Mov Disord 2008;23(5):631–40.

50. Mak MK, Wong-Yu IS, Shen X, et al. Long-term effects of exercise and physical therapy in people with Parkinson disease. Nat Rev Neurol 2017;13(11):689–703.

51. Ellis T, Boudreau JK, DeAngelis TR, et al. Barriers to exercise in people with Parkinson disease. Phys Ther 2013;93(5):628–36.

52. Mirelman A, Rochester L, Maidan I, et al. Addition of a non-immersive virtual reality component to treadmill training to reduce fall risk in older adults (V-TIME): a randomised controlled trial. Lancet 2016;388(10050):1170–82.

53. Ahlskog JE. Aerobic exercise: evidence for a direct brain effect to slow Parkinson disease progression. Mayo Clin Proc 2018;93(3):360–72.

54. Kwok JYY, Kwan JCY, Auyeung M, et al. Effects of mindfulness yoga vs stretching and resistance training exercises on anxiety and depression for people with Parkinson disease: a randomized clinical trial. JAMA Neurol 2019. https://doi.org/10.1001/jamaneurol.2019.0534.

55. Schenkman M, Moore CG, Kohrt WM, et al. Effect of high-intensity treadmill exercise on motor symptoms in patients with de novo Parkinson disease: a phase 2 randomized clinical trial. JAMA Neurol 2018;75(2):219–26.

56. Keus SH, Munneke M, Graziano M, et al. European physiotherapy guideline for Parkinson's disease. The Netherlands: KNGF/ParkinsonNet; 2014.

57. van der Marck MA, Bloem BR. How to organize multispecialty care for patients with Parkinson's disease. Parkinsonism Relat Disord 2014;20(Suppl 1):S167–73.

58. Eggers C, Dano R, Schill J, et al. Patient-centered integrated healthcare improves quality of life in Parkinson's disease patients: a randomized controlled trial. J Neurol 2018;265:764–73.

59. Ferrazzoli D, Ortelli P, Zivi I, et al. Efficacy of intensive multidisciplinary rehabilitation in Parkinson's disease: a randomised controlled study. J Neurol Neurosurg Psychiatry 2018;89(8):828–35.

60. Bloem BR, Munneke M. Revolutionising management of chronic disease: the ParkinsonNet approach. BMJ 2014;348:g1838.

61. Bloem BR, Rompen L, de Vries NM, et al. ParkinsonNet: a low cost health care innovation with a systems approach from The Netherlands. Health Aff (Millwood) 2017;36(11):1987–96.

62. Bloem BR, Munneke M. Evidence or clinical implementation: which should come first? Lancet Neurol 2014;13(7):649.

63. Nijkrake MJ, Keus SH, Overeem S, et al. The ParkinsonNet concept: development, implementation and initial experience. Mov Disord 2010;25(7):823–9.

64. Munneke M, Nijkrake MJ, Keus SH, et al. Efficacy of community-based physiotherapy networks for patients with Parkinson's disease: a cluster-randomised trial. Lancet Neurol 2010;9(1):46–54.

65. Beersen NBM, van Galen M, Huijsmans K, et al. Onderzoek naar de meerwaarde van ParkinsonNet (Research into the added value of ParkinsonNet). Zeist, Netherlands: Vektis; 2011.

66. Wensing M, van der Eijk M, Koetsenruijter J, et al. Connectedness of healthcare professionals involved in the treatment of patients with Parkinson's disease: a social networks study. Implement Sci 2011;6:67.

67. Canoy M, Faber MJ, Munneke M, et al. Hidden treasures and secret pitfalls: application of the capability approach to ParkinsonNet. J Parkinsons Dis 2015; 5(3):575–80.
68. Ketelaar NA, Munneke M, Bloem BR, et al. Recognition of physiotherapists' expertise in Parkinson's disease. BMC Health Serv Res 2013;13:430.
69. van der Eijk M, Bloem BR, Nijhuis FA, et al. Multidisciplinary collaboration in professional networks for PD a mixed-method analysis. J Parkinsons Dis 2015;5(4): 937–45.
70. Sturkenboom IH, Graff MJ, Hendriks JC, et al. Efficacy of occupational therapy for patients with Parkinson's disease: a randomised controlled trial. Lancet Neurol 2014;13(6):557–66.
71. Sturkenboom IH, Hendriks JC, Graff MJ, et al. Economic evaluation of occupational therapy in Parkinson's disease: a randomized controlled trial. Mov Disord 2015;30(8):1059–67.
72. Ypinga JHL, de Vries NM, Boonen L, et al. Effectiveness and costs of specialised physiotherapy given via ParkinsonNet: a retrospective analysis of medical claims data. Lancet Neurol 2018;17(2):153–61.
73. Maetzler W, Domingos J, Srulijes K, et al. Quantitative wearable sensors for objective assessment of Parkinson's disease. Mov Disord 2013;28(12):1628–37.
74. Rovini E, Maremmani C, Cavallo F. How wearable sensors can support Parkinson's disease diagnosis and treatment: a systematic review. Front Neurosci 2017;11:555.
75. Schneider RB, Biglan KM. The promise of telemedicine for chronic neurological disorders: the example of Parkinson's disease. Lancet Neurol 2017;16(7):541–51.
76. Broen MP, Marsman VA, Kuijf ML, et al. Unraveling the relationship between motor symptoms, affective states and contextual factors in Parkinson's disease: a feasibility study of the experience sampling method. PLoS One 2016;11(3):e0151195.
77. Mathur S, Mursaleen L, Stamford J, et al. Challenges of improving patient-centred care in Parkinson's disease. J Parkinsons Dis 2017;7(1):163–74.
78. Silva de Lima AL, Hahn T, de Vries NM, et al. Large-scale wearable sensor deployment in Parkinson's patients: the Parkinson@Home study protocol. JMIR Res Protoc 2016;5(3):e172.
79. Silva de Lima AL, Hahn T, Evers LJW, et al. Feasibility of large-scale deployment of multiple wearable sensors in Parkinson's disease. PLoS One 2017;12(12): e0189161.
80. Godinho C, Domingos J, Cunha G, et al. A systematic review of the characteristics and validity of monitoring technologies to assess Parkinson's disease. J Neuroeng Rehabil 2016;13:24.
81. Achey M, Aldred JL, Aljehani N, et al. The past, present, and future of telemedicine for Parkinson's disease. Mov Disord 2014;29(7):871–83.
82. Patel S, Chen BR, Mancinelli C, et al. Longitudinal monitoring of patients with Parkinson's disease via wearable sensor technology in the home setting. Conf Proc IEEE Eng Med Biol Soc 2011;2011:1552–5.
83. Mancini M, Bloem BR, Horak FB, et al. Clinical and methodological challenges for assessing freezing of gait: future perspectives. Mov Disord 2019. https://doi.org/10.1002/mds.27709.

Hospital Management of Parkinson Disease Patients

Adolfo Ramirez-Zamora, MD*, Takashi Tsuboi, MD, PhD

KEYWORDS

- Parkinson disease • Hospitalization • Inpatient management • Surgery • Delirium
- Falls

KEY POINTS

- Patients with Parkinson disease face a multitude of challenges during hospitalizations that requires specific management interventions.
- Management of complex dopaminergic regimens requiring frequent medication administration while hospitalized is a demanding task that can lead to errors.
- Adequate management of dopaminergic medications and avoidance of specific drugs are imperative to improve outcomes and minimize complications.
- Early implementation of fall precautions and rehabilitation therapies, including speech and swallowing assessment, is important to prevent complications and improve motor function.

INTRODUCTION

Parkinson disease (PD) is a chronic, progressive neurodegenerative disorder characterized by loss of dopaminergic cells in the substantia nigra and the accumulation of Lewy bodies. Management of PD is complex, particularly because the disease progresses and patients experience motor complications and fluctuations.[1] PD is more common in the elderly and increases in prevalence with age, and impairments in balance and coordination, falls, neuropsychiatric symptoms, swallowing difficulties, and autonomic dysfunction are prominent in later stages of the disease, increasing the risk of hospitalization. Patients with PD have more hospital admissions when compared with age- and sex-matched peers, and these admissions are associated with prolonged length of stay along with increased morbidity and mortality.[2,3]

There are a variety of causes for hospitalization, including PD-related issues ranging from elective surgeries like deep brain stimulation (DBS) to acute medical problems. Understanding the unique needs and challenges affecting this population is critical for inpatient providers and staff to provide adequate care and minimize complications.

Disclosure Statement: The authors have nothing to disclose.
University of Florida, Fixel Center for Neurological Diseases, 3009 Williston Road, Gainesville, FL 32608, USA
* Corresponding author.
E-mail address: Adolfo.Ramirez-Zamora@neurology.ufl.edu

Clin Geriatr Med 36 (2020) 173–181
https://doi.org/10.1016/j.cger.2019.09.009
0749-0690/20/© 2019 Elsevier Inc. All rights reserved.

CAUSES OF URGENT AND ELECTIVE HOSPITALIZATION IN PATIENTS WITH PARKINSON DISEASE

Prior reports regarding the frequency and the causes of hospital admissions in PD are conflicting likely because of the differences among the studied populations.[4] A systematic review noted that patients with PD are hospitalized approximately 1.5 times more frequently than non-PD patients.[5] Patients with PD (6%–45%) have an emergency room visit at least once a year, and 7% to 28% are hospitalized. In addition, international studies agree that patients with PD consistently stay in the hospital 2–14 days longer than non-PD patients.[6,7]

The International Multicenter National Parkinson Foundation Quality Improvement study initiative prospectively investigated hospitalization risks of patients with PD in PD Centers of Excellence.[8] Of 7507 patients with PD, 25.6% had a history of hospitalization within 1 year before their baseline visit. Associated hospitalization factors included race, history of DBS, utilization of physical therapy, number of comorbidities, performance on the standardized Timed Up and Go Test, and caregiver strain. Patients with a history of hospitalization before the baseline visit had a higher rate of rehospitalization. Interestingly, the time to a second hospitalization was significantly associated with caregiver burden and the number of comorbidities.[8]

The reasons for admission in PD can be categorized into the 3 following groups: (1) direct disease-related complications (eg, motor fluctuations, psychiatric symptoms, autonomic dysfunction, and side effects of dopaminergic drugs); (2) indirect disease-related complications (eg, pneumonia and trauma); and (3) systemic diseases unrelated to PD.[5] Hospitalization owing to systemic diseases might require either urgent (eg, cardiovascular and cerebrovascular diseases) or elective treatment (eg, cancers and general surgical procedures). A large retrospective study in the United States analyzed hospitalization data for more than a decade to determine the epidemiology of hospitalizations in patients with PD.[6] The mean age on admission was 78 years, and pneumonia accounted for 6.3% of PD hospitalizations, followed by urinary tract infection (4.9%), sepsis (4.5%), and aspiration pneumonitis (3.9%). Pneumonia is particularly relevant in this population, because patients with PD and parkinsonism generally develop impaired swallowing, making them susceptible to aspiration pneumonia. Other studies suggest that falls are the most common reason for hospitalization, because they occur frequently in patients with PD, leading to injury and poor quality of life (QOL).[9,10] A large population-based study in Australia suggested that people with PD were disproportionately represented among older adults hospitalized for falls.[2] Symptoms such as postural instability, orthostatic hypotension, unsteady gait, bradykinesia, and rigidity increase the risk of fall-related injuries. Additional risk factors associated with falls include age, duration of disease, difficulty performing activities of daily living, and severity of motor symptoms.[11] Research using the Medicare database also indicates that patients with PD have a higher prevalence of bone fractures and increased utilization of health care resources, particularly in the setting of fall-related injuries.[6] Finally, other common reasons for emergency admissions are infectious diseases, including aspiration pneumonia, urinary tract infection, psychiatric symptoms, medication control, and systemic disorders.[12]

CARE OF PATIENTS WITH PARKINSON DISEASE IN THE HOSPITAL SETTING

Patients with PD face a multitude of challenges during hospitalizations that required specific management interventions. **Table 1** summarizes some of the most common strategies to manage patients with PD during hospitalization.

Table 1
Common hospitalization-related issues and management approach

Regular administration of dopaminergic drugs	• Ascertain the correct medication regimen early and follow it if possible • Avoid abrupt cessation of dopaminergic drugs because this can result in severe complications, such as falls, aspiration pneumonia, or parkinsonism hyperpyrexia syndrome • If patients are unable to take drugs orally, consider using nasogastric tubes, rotigotine patches, levodopa infusion, inhaled levodopa, or subcutaneous apomorphine (if available)
Adjustment of dopaminergic medications	• Patients may need adjustment of antiparkinsonian drugs to control wearing off and dyskinesia • Dopaminergic drugs might need to be reduced in patients with dementia, psychosis, or orthostatic hypotension • If possible, avoid introducing new agents with unknown side effects
Contraindicated drugs	• Dopamine-blocking drugs, such as antipsychotics and some antiemetics (metoclopramide and prochlorperazine), should not be given because of worsening effects on motor symptoms
Delirium	• Identify and treat provoking factors, especially infections, dehydration, metabolic changes, trauma, and drugs • Remove drugs that have anticholinergic effects like benztropine and amantadine • Minimize or avoid centrally acting medications, such as narcotics, anxiolytics, hypnotics, and antidepressants • Antispasmodics for the bladder symptoms, H2 receptor antagonists, antiarrhythmic agents, antihypertensive agents, or antibiotics (cefepime) might contribute to delirium, discontinue when possible • Give frequent reorientation of the patient to the hospital environment • Consider temporarily simplifying dopaminergic regimen
Orthostatic hypotension	• Optimize hydration status • Adjust antihypertensive medications • Consider cardiac workup; tilt table test as indicated • Consider use of above the knee compression stockings • Reduce antiparkinsonian drugs if needed and possible
Management of neuropsychiatric symptoms	• Assess for intercurrent infections and consider adjustment of medications if hallucinations are present • Low-dose quetiapine might be used • Ensure adequate control of motor symptoms to prevent nonmotor wearing off • Judicious use of short-term benzodiazepine can be considered during hospital stay for severe anxiety
Patients with DBS devices	• DBS needs to be turned off during specific tests (eg, electrocardiogram) and operations using electrocautery • Consultations to movement disorder specialists and radiologists are recommended before undergoing MRI

Arguably, the most challenging task pertaining to the care of hospitalized patients with PD is management of complex medication regimens requiring frequent administration throughout the day. Many times, the hospital staff is unfamiliar with the disease and the need of precise timing of medications. Abrupt cessation of PD medications may have severe consequences, such as worsening mobility and reemergence of nonmotor symptoms. Occasionally, different levodopa formulations are used by patients throughout the day that are not interchangeable. Using a different formulation either by mistake or based on hospital availability can lead to impaired mobility because the bioavailability of carbidopa/levodopa controlled release or extended release is different[13] than the standard (immediate-release) formulation. Levodopa should be taken before or after meals to be entirely effective (this includes patients receiving tube and enteral feedings), but this is routinely omitted in hospital practice.[14] The structured hospital protocols do not allow for frequent medication dosing in PD. An algorithm for estimating parenteral doses of dopaminergic drugs in perioperative settings has been proposed.[15]

Although issues related to the administration of medications have not been systematically studied, several reports illustrate the challenges of administering medications correctly during hospitalizations. In 1 study that audited medication administration for patients with PD with hospitalizations greater than 48 hours, medication errors included missed doses of PD medications (48%) and delayed administration of medications by more than 30 minutes (44%).[16] This study also found that 21% of patients received medications that are considered contraindicated in those with PD. These errors are consistent with concerns raised by surveys completed by patients and caregivers.[17] A Hospitalization Kit has been developed by the Parkinson's Foundation to bring attention to these issues (https://www.parkinson.org/Living-with-Parkinsons/Resources-and-Support/Patient-Safety-Kit). The kits have information to provide the inpatient medical staff.

Long delays for restarting levodopa should be avoided because this may result in a loss of previous adequate duration of levodopa response, particularly in the setting of recent surgery and anesthesia. Abrupt cessation of antiparkinsonian medications can lead to the development of Parkinsonism-hyperpyrexia syndrome or a dopamine agonist withdrawal syndrome. It is important to allow administration of PD medications during the nothing-by-mouth status with timely utilization of nasogastric tubes in hospitalized patients with PD with compromised swallowing function. Orally dissolving formulations of levodopa are available in some hospitals, which can be used until enteral feedings are established.

Dyskinesia are involuntary choreoathetoid or dystonic movements associated with the use of levodopa in PD. Dyskinesia can jeopardize orthopedic procedures and wound healing and increase the risk of falls. These movements commonly occur during peak medication effect, and judicious reduction of dopaminergic doses can be instituted.

Patients with PD might experience orthostatic hypotension (OH), increasing their risk of falls or syncope. During hospitalizations, the risk of OH increases in instances of hypovolemia related to recent surgery, nothing-by-mouth status, blood loss, diarrhea, prolonged bed rest, and the use of antihypertensive drugs or diuretics. Evaluating for OH is critical in different positions (supine and standing). Initial strategies for management include nonpharmacologic treatments (ie, compression stockings and exercises), restoring euvolemia, and cessation of offending drugs. The use of medications, such as fludrocortisone, droxidopa, and midodrine, should be considered carefully because of potential side effects, including supine hypertension.[18]

Insomnia is a common problem in patients with PD that frequently worsens during hospital stays. Levodopa doses need to be administered commonly at night to prevent nocturnal bradykinesia, but other reasons for insomnia include nocturia, sleep apnea, delirium, and reversal of sleep and wake cycle. Addressing each concern specifically is needed to improve sleep. The use of hypnotics is acceptable, but caution should be used with benzodiazepines.

Patients with PD are at an increased risk for delirium in the hospital, and management should include a review and adjustment of medications with centrally acting properties, early recognition, reduction of sleep disruptions, maintenance of a stable hospital room, prompt treatment of infection, as well as frequent reorientation of the patient to the hospital environment.[19] Patients with PD are 5 times more likely to be treated for delirium and 3 times more likely to experience an adverse drug event and syncope.[2] The cause of delirium is usually multifactorial, including metabolic, toxic, or infectious causes, with a risk for postoperative delirium varying 2.8% and 8.1% among patients with PD compared with controls.[20]

Hallucinations and psychosis might occur during hospitalizations, and reduction of dopaminergic medications is occasionally required, specifically dopamine agonists because they are more likely to provoke psychosis.[21] Other drugs that can be discontinued include amantadine or monoamine oxidase B (MAO-B) inhibitors with long half-lives. The use of quetiapine or clozapine can be considered.[18] Quetiapine can be started in a single dose at night with gradual dose increases guided by clinical benefit. Pimavanserin, a recently approved drug for PD psychosis, has not been studied in the inpatient setting, and there is a delay of weeks before an observed clinical benefit in symptoms, which limits its use in the hospital.

Nausea is common during hospitalizations, but the antiemetic medications metoclopramide and prochlorperazine that block dopamine should be avoided because of an increased risk of worsening parkinsonism. Acceptable alternative medications include ondansetron and trimethobenzamide.

Pain management is another challenging aspect of PD management during hospitalizations. Patients with PD experience different types of pain related to the disease, surgical procedures, or systemic problems. Narcotics should be used cautiously because of centrally depressing properties and risk of worsening nonmotor symptoms. It is important to recognize dystonic or musculoskeletal pain, which is usually related to worsening parkinsonism and may promptly respond to adjustments in levodopa dose.

Management of medications calls for an interdisciplinary approach, including patient, caregiver, nurse, treating physician, pharmacist, along with patient's treating neurologist to optimize medical management during hospitalization.

PERIOPERATIVE CARE

As life expectancy continues to increase, an increasing number of patients with PD undergo elective or emergent surgeries. In a nationwide database study from Taiwan that assessed postoperative complications between 6455 patients with PD and 12,910 non-PD patients who underwent major surgeries, patients with PD had a higher risk of postoperative pulmonary embolism (odds ratio [OR] 2.72), pneumonia (OR 1.98), stroke (OR 1.77), septicemia (OR 1.54), urinary tract infection (OR 1.52), acute renal failure (OR 1.36), and mortality (OR 1.45).[22] Similar results from other countries have been reported in patients with PD who underwent orthopedic surgeries.[23,24]

All the antiparkinsonian medications except for MAO-B inhibitors should be continued as long as possible before surgery. MOA-B inhibitors are desirable to be discontinued 1 to 2 weeks before surgery to minimize the risk of medication interactions.[25] These medications may contribute to intraoperative fluctuations in blood pressure and also increase the risk of serotonin syndrome. In addition, interactions with opioids, especially meperidine, have been reported. If the patients are receiving DBS, consultation to movement disorder specialists before surgery is indicated to ensure that appropriate precautions are taken regarding specific surgical procedures and imaging studies.

Regional anesthesia may be preferable to general anesthesia in terms of postoperative nausea and vomiting.[26] In general, less invasive interventions, such as laparoscopic rather than open surgeries, are recommended given faster postoperative recovery. On the other hand, general anesthesia may be a better choice for patients with marked dyskinesia, because these movements can interfere with the surgical procedure. It is important to note that propofol can exacerbate dyskinesia.[26] Fentanyl should be avoided because of potential worsening effects on parkinsonian motor symptoms.[25]

After surgery, medications for PD management should be resumed as soon as possible (using a nasogastric tube if needed as pointed out in earlier discussion), which may reduce the risks of complications, such as aspiration pneumonia, pulmonary embolisms due to immobility, and falls.

In routine clinical practice, antidopaminergic drugs, such as antipsychotics (typical and atypical neuroleptics), and antiemetics (metoclopramide and prochlorperazine) are frequently prescribed for postoperative psychiatric symptoms and gastrointestinal problems, respectively. However, these drugs should not be administrated to patients with PD because they worsen motor symptoms and are potentially life threatening. Finally, earlier intervention with rehabilitation and speech and swallowing services may be beneficial for preventing complications and promoting recovery.

STRATEGIES TO MINIMIZE HOSPITALIZATION IN PARKINSON DISEASE

Additional strategies and early interventions have been suggested to maintain mobility and complications and reduce falls and fractures in people with PD (**Table 2**). Education is paramount, and a recent study conducted by the National Parkinson Foundation reported an increased need for education and communication among hospitalists and hospital staff to reduce inpatient admissions.[27] Early identification of impaired swallowing function might allow earlier initiation of interventions to treat or prevent aspiration pneumonia. Promising evidence supports improving access to outpatient clinics as an essential strategy to minimize hospitalizations, complications, and prolonged hospital stays.[19] Addressing avoidable medication errors is critical, and engaging patients and caregivers might reduce these concerns and improve quality of inpatient care.[28]

PALLIATIVE CARE

Palliative care is a specialty that focuses on improving QOL for patients with serious diseases and their families. Primary palliative care skills may be particularly relevant to clinicians who see patients with chronic neurologic diseases, including PD, because of the complexity of their clinical symptoms.

As the disease progresses, patients with PD experience various symptoms, which are often difficult to control. In a study on 129 pathologically proven patients with PD, the following milestones are indicated: visual hallucinations preceded death by 5.1 years; regular falls by 4.1 years; dementia by 3.3 years; and need for residential care by 3.3 years.[29] Importantly, the older the age at onset, the earlier the patient had the milestones mentioned above. Thus, hospitalizations because of direct or indirect disease-related complications can be an opportunity to introduce palliative care, although palliative care is appropriate even at the time of diagnosis. Establishing goals of care to relieve symptoms and maximize overall QOL may be of central importance at the advanced stage. Establishing clear goals for treatment and prioritizing treatment of specific symptoms by patients and their families are imperative. A multidisciplinary

Table 2
Preventive strategies to minimize complications during hospitalization in patients with Parkinson disease

General admission tips	• Advise patients/caregivers to always carry up-to-date medication list • Confirm correct levodopa formulation to avoid confusion or unwanted substitutions • Observe appropriate timing of levodopa related to meals, surgical times, and bedtime • Educate the primary medical team and nursing staff on the importance of timely administration of medications • Consult neurology early during hospitalization course • Provide consistent emotional support and adequate sleep hygiene • Avoiding prolonged naps during the day
Ensure adequate administration of dopaminergic medications drugs	• See above • PD medications should be administered as closely to home schedule as possible
Falls and fracture prevention	• Implement fall preventions, bisphosphonates, vitamin D supplementation • Start physical therapy and assistive devices • Obtain bone density scans
Rehabilitation	• Mobilize patients as much and as early as possible to maintain/improve motor function and to prevent falls and deep vein thrombosis (DVT) • Consider swallowing rehabilitation to reduce the risk of aspiration pneumonia • Minimize aspiration risk (chin-down swallow, expiratory muscle strength training, education)
Possible complications during hospitalization	• Monitor closely for signs of complications suggesting pneumonia, urinary tract infections, DVT, gastrointestinal, or electrolyte disturbances • Administer pulmonary toileting • Ensure sufficient nutritional intake and treat constipation early and aggressively • Monitor for the development of paralytic ileus in patients with abdominal surgery and treat accordingly. Case reports suggest potential use of prokinetic agents prophylactically • Implement regular turning in bed to prevent pressure sores • Ensure adequate fluid intake
Perioperative management	• Arrange for a surgery early in the day • Continue dopaminergic drugs until the morning of surgery and resume as soon as possible postoperatively • Consider nonoral formulations (rotigotine patches, inhaled levodopa, or subcutaneous apomorphine) or orally dissolving levodopa if needed • Regional anesthesia allows monitoring of Parkinson symptoms and might be best in patients who require very frequent dopaminergic medications
Minimizing need of hospitalizations	• Early neurology consultation • Open access clinics and compliance with PD medication might reduce hospital admissions and emergency room visits by patients with PD.

care team involving physicians, nurses, rehabilitation therapists, and other health care providers may further improve QOL.

REFERENCES

1. Okun MS. Management of Parkinson disease in 2017: personalized approaches for patient-specific needs. JAMA 2017;318(9):791–2.
2. Lubomski M, Rushworth RL, Tisch S. Hospitalisation and comorbidities in Parkinson's disease: a large Australian retrospective study. J Neurol Neurosurg Psychiatry 2015;86(3):324–30.
3. Aminoff MJ, Christine CW, Friedman JH, et al. Management of the hospitalized patient with Parkinson's disease: current state of the field and need for guidelines. Parkinsonism Relat Disord 2011;17(3):139–45.
4. Oguh O, Videnovic A. Inpatient management of Parkinson disease: current challenges and future directions. Neurohospitalist 2012;2(1):28–35.
5. Gerlach OH, Winogrodzka A, Weber WE. Clinical problems in the hospitalized Parkinson's disease patient: systematic review. Mov Disord 2011;26(2):197–208.
6. Mahajan A, Balakrishnan P, Patel A, et al. Epidemiology of inpatient stay in Parkinson's disease in the United States: insights from the nationwide inpatient sample. J Clin Neurosci 2016;31:162–5.
7. Kelly B, Blake C, Lennon O. Acute hospital admissions of individuals with a known Parkinson's disease diagnosis in Ireland 2009-2012: a short report. J Parkinsons Dis 2016;6(4):709–16.
8. Shahgholi L, De Jesus S, Wu SS, et al. Hospitalization and rehospitalization in Parkinson disease patients: data from the National Parkinson Foundation Centers of Excellence. PLoS One 2017;12(7):e0180425.
9. Martignoni E, Godi L, Citterio A, et al. Comorbid disorders and hospitalisation in Parkinson's disease: a prospective study. Neurol Sci 2004;25(2):66–71.
10. Paul SS, Harvey L, Canning CG, et al. Fall-related hospitalization in people with Parkinson's disease. Eur J Neurol 2017;24(3):523–9.
11. Cheng KY, Lin WC, Chang WN, et al. Factors associated with fall-related fractures in Parkinson's disease. Parkinsonism Relat Disord 2014;20(1):88–92.
12. Fujioka S, Fukae J, Ogura H, et al. Hospital-based study on emergency admission of patients with Parkinson's disease. eNeurologicalSci 2016;4:19–21.
13. Ahlskog JE, Muenter MD, McManis PG, et al. Controlled-release Sinemet (CR-4): a double-blind crossover study in patients with fluctuating Parkinson's disease. Mayo Clin Proc 1988;63(9):876–86.
14. Magdalinou KN, Martin A, Kessel B. Prescribing medications in Parkinson's disease (PD) patients during acute admissions to a District General Hospital. Parkinsonism Relat Disord 2007;13(8):539–40.
15. Brennan KA, Genever RW. Managing Parkinson's disease during surgery. BMJ 2010;341:c5718.
16. Wu L, WS, Moore J, et al. Assessment of medical care for patients with Parkinson's disease during hospitalization. Mov Disord 2009;24:S378–9.
17. Buetow S, Henshaw J, Bryant L, et al. Medication timing errors for Parkinson's disease: perspectives held by caregivers and people with Parkinson's in New Zealand. Parkinsons Dis 2010;2010:432983.
18. Seppi K, Ray Chaudhuri K, Coelho M, et al. Update on treatments for nonmotor symptoms of Parkinson's disease–an evidence-based medicine review. Mov Disord 2019;34(2):180–98.

19. Klein C, Prokhorov T, Miniovitz A, et al. Admission of Parkinsonian patients to a neurological ward in a community hospital. J Neural Transm (Vienna) 2009; 116(11):1509–12.
20. Golden WE, Lavender RC, Metzer WS. Acute postoperative confusion and hallucinations in Parkinson disease. Ann Intern Med 1989;111(3):218–22.
21. Parkinson Study G. Pramipexole vs levodopa as initial treatment for Parkinson disease: a randomized controlled trial. Parkinson Study Group. JAMA 2000; 284(15):1931–8.
22. Huang YF, Chou YC, Yeh CC, et al. Outcomes after non-neurological surgery in patients with Parkinson's disease: a nationwide matched cohort study. Medicine (Baltimore) 2016;95(12):e3196.
23. Newman JM, Sodhi N, Wilhelm AB, et al. Parkinson's disease increases the risk of perioperative complications after total knee arthroplasty: a nationwide database study. Knee Surg Sports Traumatol Arthrosc 2018;27(7):2189–95.
24. McClelland S 3rd, Baker JF, Smith JS, et al. Impact of Parkinson's disease on perioperative complications and hospital cost in multilevel spine fusion: a population-based analysis. J Clin Neurosci 2017;35:88–91.
25. Burton DA, Nicholson G, Hall GM. Anaesthesia in elderly patients with neurodegenerative disorders: special considerations. Drugs Aging 2004;21(4):229–42.
26. Nicholson G, Pereira AC, Hall GM. Parkinson's disease and anaesthesia. Br J Anaesth 2002;89(6):904–16.
27. Chou KL, Zamudio J, Schmidt P, et al. Hospitalization in Parkinson disease: a survey of National Parkinson Foundation centers. Parkinsonism Relat Disord 2011; 17(6):440–5.
28. Gerlach OH, Broen MP, Weber WE. Motor outcomes during hospitalization in Parkinson's disease patients: a prospective study. Parkinsonism Relat Disord 2013; 19(8):737–41.
29. Kempster PA, O'Sullivan SS, Holton JL, et al. Relationships between age and late progression of Parkinson's disease: a clinico-pathological study. Brain 2010; 133(Pt 6):1755–62.

Moving?

Make sure your subscription moves with you!

To notify us of your new address, find your **Clinics Account Number** (located on your mailing label above your name), and contact customer service at:

Email: journalscustomerservice-usa@elsevier.com

800-654-2452 (subscribers in the U.S. & Canada)
314-447-8871 (subscribers outside of the U.S. & Canada)

Fax number: 314-447-8029

Elsevier Health Sciences Division
Subscription Customer Service
3251 Riverport Lane
Maryland Heights, MO 63043

*To ensure uninterrupted delivery of your subscription,
please notify us at least 4 weeks in advance of move.

Printed and bound by CPI Group (UK) Ltd, Croydon, CR0 4YY

03/10/2024

01040406-0020